Clinical Management of Cardiovascular Risk Factors in Diabetes

Second Edition

Marvin Moser, MD, FACP
Clinical Professor of Medicine
Yale University School of Medicine

James R. Sowers, MD
Professor of Medicine, Physiology, and Pharmacology
University of Missouri–Columbia

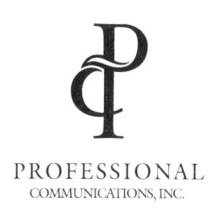

PROFESSIONAL
COMMUNICATIONS, INC.

Copyright 2005
Marvin Moser, MD and
James R. Sowers, MD

Professional Communications, Inc.
A Medical Publishing Company

Marketing Office:
400 Center Bay Drive
West Islip, NY 11795
(t) 631/661-2852
(f) 631/661-2167

Editorial Office:
PO Box 10
Caddo, OK 74729-0010
(t) 580/367-9838
(f) 580/367-9989

All rights reserved. No part of this publication may be reproduced or transmitted in any form or by any means, electronic or mechanical, including photocopy, recording, or any other information storage and retrieval system, without the prior agreement and written permission of the publisher.

For orders only, please call
1-800-337-9838
or visit our website at
www.pcibooks.com

ISBN: 1-932610-01-4

Printed in the United States of America

DISCLAIMER
The opinions expressed in this publication reflect those of the authors. However, the authors make no warranty regarding the contents of the publication. The protocols described herein are general and may not apply to a specific patient. Any product mentioned in this publication should be taken in accordance with the prescribing information provided by the manufacturer.

This text is printed on recycled paper.

DEDICATION

To our colleagues and students who are working to reduce the cardiovascular consequences of diabetes, hypertension, and dyslipidemia. In this era of interventional and procedure-driven medicine, it is important to be reminded by them of the important contributions that good patient care and attention to risk-factor modification can play in preventing cardiovascular disease.

ACKNOWLEDGMENT

We express our gratitude to Adrienne Cramer and Paddy McGowan, who have worked with us as research and administrative assistants for many years, and to Malcolm Beasley and Phyllis Freeny for their guidance and help in editing the manuscript. Finally, our thanks to the Hypertension Education Foundation, Inc. for research support.

TABLE OF CONTENTS

Part 1 *Epidemiology and Scope of Problem*	Introduction	1
	Diabetes in the United States	2
	Scope of and Risk Factors for Cardiovascular Disease in Diabetic Patients	3
Part 2 *Cardiovascular Disease in Diabetics*	Pathophysiologic/Metabolic Interactions Between Diabetes and Cardiovascular Disease	4
	The Renin-Angiotensin-Aldosterone System in Diabetes	5
Part 3 *Management of Hypertension*	Results of Hypertension Treatment Trials in Diabetic Patients	6
Part 4 *Management Approaches to Cardiovascular Risk Reduction in Diabetes*	Cardiovascular Risk Reduction in Hypertensive Diabetics	7
	Cardiovascular Risk Reduction: Lipid-Lowering Therapy	8
	Cardiovascular Risk Reduction: Antiplatelet Therapy	9
	Cardiovascular Risk Reduction: Control of Diabetes	10
	Risk Reduction in Special Populations	11
	Target Organs and Diabetes	12
Part 5 *Summary and Index*	Summary of Cardiovascular Disease Reduction in Diabetics	13
	Index	14

TABLES

Table 2.1	Metabolic and Cardiovascular Risk Factors Associated With Visceral Obesity	26
Table 2.2	Criteria for Testing for Diabetes in Asymptomatic, Undiagnosed Individuals	27
Table 2.3	Criteria for the Diagnosis of Diabetes Mellitus	28
Table 3.1	Definitions of Abnormalities in Albumin Excretion	36
Table 3.2	Clinical Features of the Metabolic Syndrome	40
Table 4.1	Lipoprotein Abnormalities in Patients With Hypertension as Well as in Those With Diabetes Mellitus	47
Table 4.2	Hemodynamic Characteristics of Hypertension in Diabetes	53
Table 4.3	Some of the Alterations in Vascular Endothelium Associated With Diabetes and Hypertension	57
Table 4.4	Coagulation and Fibrinolytic Abnormalities in Diabetes and Hypertension	58
Table 4.5	Platelet Function Abnormalities in Diabetes and Hypertension	59
Table 4.6	Cardiovascular Risk Factors That Tend to Cluster With Microalbuminuria	62
Table 4.7	Microalbuminuria	70
Table 5.1	Effects of Moderate- and High-Dose Diuretic Therapy on Glucose Metabolism in Placebo-Controlled Trials	80
Table 5.2	New-Onset Diabetes in the Prospective, Comparative, Randomized Hypertension Treatment Trials (3-to-8 Years Follow-Up)	82
Table 5.3	Incidence of New-Onset Diabetes With Different Antihypertensive Medications in the 3-to-8 Year Hypertension Treatment Trials	86
Table 6.1	Hypertension Detection and Follow-Up Program Results in Diabetic Subjects	93
Table 6.2	Cumulative 5-Year Rates (1000 Patient Years) of Cardiovascular Events in the Systolic Hypertension in the Elderly Program	96

Table 6.3	Symptoms in Active-Therapy Diabetic Subjects Compared With Placebo Subjects in the Systolic Hypertension in the Elderly Program	99
Table 6.4	Major Outcome Events in Patients With Type 1 Diabetes and Nephropathy	102
Table 6.5	Baseline Characteristics of Patients With Diabetic Nephropathy in the Captopril and Placebo Groups	103
Table 6.6	Adjusted Cardiovascular Events in the Appropriate Blood Pressure Control in Diabetes Study	105
Table 6.7	Cardiovascular Events in the Fosinopril vs Amlodipine Cardiovascular Events Trial	106
Table 6.8	Results of Different Levels of Blood Pressure Control in Hypertensive Patients With Type 2 Diabetes: β-Blocker Compared With ACE Inhibitor–Based Treatment Program	109
Table 6.9	United Kingdom Prospective Diabetes Study: Effect of Blood Pressure Control on Diabetic Events	110
Table 6.10	Risk Reduction in Diabetic Subjects in the Captopril Prevention Project (CAPPP)	115
Table 6.11	Systolic Hypertension in the Elderly Trial: Results in Diabetics	116
Table 6.12	Results of the Heart Outcome Prevention Evaluation Study in Diabetes	131
Table 6.13	Randomized Controlled Clinical Trials of Antihypertensive Therapy in Type 2 Diabetic Patients With Hypertension	132
Table 6.14	Answers Provided by the Treatment Trials in Diabetics With Hypertension	136
Table 7.1	Lifestyle Modifications for Control of Hypertension and/or Overall Cardiovascular Risk	143
Table 7.2	Risk Stratification of Hypertension to Guide Treatment Choices	144
Table 7.3	Lifestyle Modifications	145
Table 7.4	Calculating Body Mass Index and Desirable Ranges	147

Table 7.5	Simple Method of Calculating Ideal Weight	148
Table 7.6	Calculating Calories to Maintain or Lose Weight	148
Table 7.7	Some High–Sodium-Content Foods That Should Be Avoided	149
Table 7.8	ACE Inhibitors Used for Treating Hypertension	154
Table 7.9	Angiotensin II Receptor Blockers Used for Treating Hypertension	157
Table 7.10	Some Commonly Used Diuretics for Treating Hypertension	159
Table 7.11	GEMINI Study: Comparison of Carvedilol and Metoprolol in Diabetic Patients	162
Table 7.12	β-Blockers and Combined α_1/β-Blocker Used for Treating Hypertension	164
Table 7.13	Combination Antihypertensive Medications	168
Table 8.1	Diet Recommendations for the Treatment of Lipid Disorders in Diabetes	178
Table 8.2	Lipid-Lowering Drugs: Preparations and Usual Dosing Regimens	182
Table 8.3	Reduction in Nonfatal MI or CAD Death in Patients With Diabetes Mellitus and CAD in Clinical Trials	186
Table 8.4	Guidelines for Lipid-Lowering Therapy in Patients With Diabetes	195
Table 8.5	Order of Priorities for Treatment of Diabetic Dyslipidemia in Adults	197
Table 8.6	Medications for the Treatment of Dyslipidemia in Adults	198
Table 8.7	Efficacy of HMG-CoA Reductase Inhibitors	199
Table 10.1	Glycemic Control in People With Diabetes	209
Table 10.2	Nutritional Goals, Principles, and Recommendations	212
Table 10.3	Precautions for Diabetic Patients With Medical Complications	215
Table 10.4	Guidelines for Safe Exercise	216

Table 10.5	Warning Symptoms and Signs of Diabetic Foot Problems	219
Table 10.6	Characteristics of Currently Available Oral Antidiabetic Agents	222
Table 13.1	Guide to Prevention of Cardiovascular Disease in Patients With Diabetes	252

FIGURES

Figure 2.1	Estimated Number of Adults Worldwide With Diabetes by Age Group and Year	20
Figure 2.2	Prevalence of Diabetes Among People ≥20 Years of Age: United States, 2002	21
Figure 2.3	Age-Specific Prevalence of Diagnosed Diabetes by Race/Ethnicity and Gender: United States, 2002	22
Figure 2.4	United Kingdom Prospective Diabetic Study: Epidemiology	23
Figure 2.5	Diabetes Reduces Years of Life	24
Figure 2.6	Increase in Prevalence of Obesity Over the Past Decade (%)	25
Figure 3.1	Risk of Cardiovascular Events in Type 2 Diabetes	35
Figure 3.2	Association of Systolic Blood Pressure and Cardiovascular Death in Type 2 Diabetes	41
Figure 4.1	Pathogenesis of Hypertension in the Insulin-Resistant State	50
Figure 4.2	ACE Inhibition	51
Figure 4.3	Relationship of Elevated Systolic Blood Pressure and Complications of Diabetes	52
Figure 4.4	24-Hour Systolic Blood Pressure Measurements	54
Figure 4.5	Microalbuminuria and Ischemic Heart Disease Risk	61
Figure 4.6	Association of Microalbuminuria and Cardiovascular Morbidity and Mortality in Type 2 Diabetes	69

Figure 5.1	Site of Action of ACE Inhibitors and Angiotensin II Receptor Blockers	74
Figure 6.1	Systolic Hypertension in the Elderly Program: Influence of Diabetes on Cardiovascular Event Rates	95
Figure 6.2	Morbidity and Mortality in Diabetic and Nondiabetic Subjects in the Systolic Hypertension in the Elderly Program	97
Figure 6.3	United Kingdom Prospective Diabetes Study	108
Figure 6.4	Results of Tight Blood Pressure Control Compared With Less-Tight Blood Pressure Control in United Kingdom Prospective Diabetes Study	112
Figure 6.5	Comparison of Captopril–Based and β-Blocker/Diuretic–Based Therapy in Patients With Diabetes in the Captopril Prevention Project (CAPPP)	114
Figure 6.6	Relative Risk of Elevated Systolic and Diastolic Blood Pressure	118
Figure 6.7	Patients With Diabetes in the Hypertension Optimal Treatment Trial	120
Figure 6.8	Cardiovascular Events in Diabetics in the Hypertension Optimal Treatment Study	121
Figure 6.9	Kaplan-Meier Curves of the Percentage of Type 2 Diabetic Patients With End-Stage Renal Disease in the RENAAL Study	124
Figure 6.10	Cumulative Proportions of Patients Reaching Primary End Points in the IDNT	126
Figure 6.11	Progression of Diabetic Nephropathy in IRMA 2 Study of Hypertensive Patients With Type 2 Diabetes and Microproteinuria	128
Figure 6.12	Clinical Outcomes Among Diabetic Hypertensives Treated With Losartan or Atenolol in the LIFE Study	130
Figure 7.1	Suggested Treatment Program for Patients With Hypertension and Type 2 Diabetes	140
Figure 7.2	Risk of Hyperglycemia With Use of Antihypertensive Drugs	161
Figure 7.3	Major Cardiovascular Events According to Treatment	167

Figure 8.1	Simvastatin vs Placebo: Curves for Probability of Remaining Free of a Major Coronary Heart Disease Event 185
Figure 8.2	Effect of Pravastatin on Relative Risks of Cardiovascular Events in Patients With or Without Clinically Diagnosed Diabetes 188
Figure 8.3	Effects of Simvastatin Therapy Compared With Placebo on First Major Vascular Event in Different Prior Disease Categories 190
Figure 8.4	Changes in Lipid Values From Baseline in Placebo and Fenofibrate Groups 192
Figure 10.1	Treatment Algorithm for Glycemic Control of Type 2 Diabetes 226

PREFACE TO SECOND EDITION

Both diabetes and hypertension are on the increase in the United States, in part related to increased obesity and the aging of our population. The coexistence of diabetes and hypertension is also increasingly common, and patients with both disorders are at a considerably higher risk for cardiovascular disease (CVD) than individuals with either disease alone. This updated text addresses current knowledge and guidelines in the prevention and treatment of CVD in patients with coexisting diabetes and hypertension. In addition, it reviews newer data on the management of dyslipidemia and nephropathy in diabetic patients. A clear message emerges—several major risk factors that adversely impact the life of patients with the metabolic syndrome and/or diabetes can be controlled and lives prolonged if these risk factors are controlled.

1 Introduction

The history of the prevention of heart attack, stroke, and heart failure by altering known cardiovascular (CV) risk factors is an exciting one. Perhaps nowhere else has such an impact been made in preventive medicine other than in the prevention of infectious diseases, such as typhoid fever and polio, by the use of vaccines. Interventions to prevent vascular diseases followed the recognition of various factors that increased the risk for cardiovascular disease (CVD). These included hypertension, smoking, and hyperlipidemia. A disease that appears to cluster with many of these factors is diabetes. Most diabetic patients:

- Have elevated blood pressure (BP)
- Are obese
- Have hyperlipidemia
- Have coagulation disorders.

Any one of these specific entities poses a risk for an increase in CV events. When these risk factors occur in conjunction with diabetes, CVD risk is considerably increased.

Until recent years, most efforts in managing diabetes concentrated on glycemic control with diet, insulin, or antidiabetic medications. Most of the studies designed to show that tight control of blood glucose levels would reduce CV events in type 2 diabetic patients have proven to be only marginally successful. With extremely tight glycemic control, some success has been noted in preventing the microvascular complications of diabetes (ie, retinopathy, neuropathy, renal disease, etc), but effects on CV end points have not been consistently demonstrated. Too many diabetic patients are unable or unwilling to alter their lifestyle enough or to take the appropriate medication to bring about this degree of blood glucose control required to prevent complications. In addition, there are problems with weight gain and hypoglycemic episodes with very tight glycemic control. In recent years, more attention has been focused on interventions to control the other risk factors that occur in the diabetic: the bottom line is that controlling hyperglycemia should only be one part of the effort of a multifaceted approach to reduce vascular complications in diabetic patients.

Hypertension, defined as a persistent BP >140/90 mm Hg, is common in diabetics. It is well recognized that the presence of hypertension in a diabetic patient greatly increases risk not only for CVD but for eye disease and renal failure. It has been known for years that a diabetic patient is at much greater risk for coronary heart disease (CHD) events than a nondiabetic with similar BP. Yet, until recently, careful management of elevated BP has not been emphasized.

The effort to control hypertension has been hindered by a variety of myths and misconceptions. Some of these relate to the following:

- Preoccupation with protecting the kidneys in patients with diabetes. It is recognized that diabetic nephropathy is common and that end-stage renal disease is a fairly frequent and serious outcome in diabetic patients. But most of the deaths that occur prematurely in diabetic patients are secondary to CVD and not renal failure. Treatment to prevent renal disease is of great importance, but as much or more emphasis should be placed on CV outcomes.
- The fact that doubt had been placed in the mind of many physicians about the potential theoretic hazards associated with the use of various antihypertensive drugs, specifically, diuretics and

β-blockers. These agents were, until recent years, the antihypertensive medications used as initial therapy in all hypertension-treatment clinical trials. Despite the fact that they were effective antihypertensive agents and that their use reduced morbidity and mortality, there were still many physicians who were reluctant to use them because of concerns about changes in insulin resistance, blood glucose, lipid levels, and the occurrence of new-onset (incipient) diabetes.
- Questions regarding the safety of another class of antihypertensive medications, the calcium channel blockers, in the management of hypertension.
- Debates about the appropriate BP level at which treatment should be started.
- Concerns about the target to which BP should be lowered. This also delayed a more aggressive approach to the management of hypertension in the patient with diabetes.

Many of these misconceptions have been clarified by results of recent clinical trials. The trials have shown that lowering of BP in diabetic patients, especially in those with non–insulin-dependent (type 2), will reduce CV events, stroke, and progression of renal disease to a greater degree than the control of elevated blood glucose levels.

This is not to conclude that glycemic control is not important—it is to emphasize that treatment programs focused only on glycemic control in such patients are no longer appropriate. All classes of currently available antihypertensive agents are safe and effective in this population. There are some outcome differences, however, which will be discussed and some preferences for specific therapy.

Treatment with lifestyle modifications and antihypertensive medications should be started earlier in a diabetic hypertensive patient than in a nondiabetic and pursued to BP levels lower than those in the nondiabetic, ie, to levels <130/80-85 mm Hg (see Chapter 4, *Pathophysiologic/Metabolic Interactions Between Diabetes and Cardiovascular Disease*, and Chapter 5, *The Renin-Angiotensin-Aldosterone System in Diabetes*). Recent data suggest that the lowest risk is associated with a systolic BP ≤120 mm Hg. Not only does BP control reduce macrovascular complications (eg, coronary events, heart failure, and stroke), but also microvascular events (eg, retinopathy and proteinuria). As this evidence has emerged from numerous trials, as well as evidence that controlling lipid levels in the diabetic patient is also beneficial, more emphasis has been placed on evaluating the diabetic patient as a panoply of the metabolic and CVD states wrapped in a diagnosis of diabetes. The conglomerate includes hyperglycemia, hyperlipidemia, hypertension, and enhanced coagulation.

Diabetes is a common disease, occurring in approximately 10% of adults in the United States. Hypertension is even more common; >50% of people >55 years of age have elevated BP defined as >140/90 mm Hg. Hyperlipidemia and obesity are present in >40% of adults in the United States.

Numerous textbooks and monographs have been written about the management of hypertension and hyperlipidemia. There is a plethora of books dealing with the dietary and drug management of the diabetic individual. *Clinical Management of Cardiovascular Risk Factors in Diabetes* is an attempt to put the data together and to outline a practical approach to the management of all of the CV risk factors in an individual with diabetes. The second edition updates recent trials, outcome studies, and guidelines that confirm a multifaceted approach to reduce CVD in this high-risk population. It is appropriate to do this so that health care providers may approach the diabetic patient not only as someone in need of dietary guidance, insulin, or other medications to control blood glucose levels, but as a patient with a complex of factors that can be treated with the expectation that morbidity/mortality will be significantly reduced.

Good data from recent prospective, randomized clinical trials are finally available so that specific recommendations can be made. These trials have demonstrated the benefits of antihypertensive, antiplatelet, and antilipid therapy in diabetic patients. Many of the misconceptions that have limited the use of therapeutic agents in hypertension have been put to rest.

Specific problems relating to hypertensive diabetic patients that may influence the choices of therapy are discussed in *Clinical Management of Cardiovascular Risk Factors in Diabetes*. These unique issues include the facts that diabetic patients often:

- Present with postural hypotension secondary to autonomic neuropathy
- Have a relatively high incidence of sexual dysfunction
- Have subclinical evidence of renal disease, ie, low levels of proteinuria
- Experience "silent" myocardial infarction and a high incidence of subclinical CVD.

Clinical Management of Cardiovascular Risk Factors in Diabetes is not intended to be a textbook. It is intended to:

- Update data on the pathophysiology of diabetes, especially as these relate to part of a clinical syndrome
- Review the specific treatments of elevated blood glucose levels, dyslipidemia, elevated BP, and coagulation abnormalities in the diabetic patient
- Summarize recent and older clinical trials that have established benefits of treatment

- Present a specific outline of treatment recommendations for the diabetic patient with or without some of the other comorbid conditions. This book presents the practitioner with a guideline based on firm scientific evidence. Special problems will be discussed in some detail with specific suggestions as to how they should be handled in the typical diabetic patient.

This second edition reviews recent trials and the new guidelines and how they can be implemented by the practicing physician.

An optimistic picture can be painted for most patients with diabetes, whether they have type 1 diabetes, a disease that once was almost universally fatal by 35 to 40 years of age, or type 2 diabetes, which often does not manifest itself until the patient is middle-aged or older. Type 1 diabetics live longer and less-confining lives with modern therapy; individuals with type 2 diabetes can now look forward to life with considerably less fear of morbid events, such as stroke and heart failure, that were once almost expected outcomes. Serious nephropathy and retinopathy can also be delayed or possibly prevented. These events may still occur but with rigorous treatment of hypertension and hyperlipidemia, as well as of the diabetes, they are considerably less common. The earlier the diabetic patient is treated, the greater the chance of preventing one of these morbid or mortal CV events.

It is our aim that this book will give the reader a guide to the clinical management of CV risk factors in diabetic patients.

2 Diabetes in the United States

Prevalence and Trends

Diabetes is a metabolic disease characterized by hyperglycemia resulting from defects in insulin action, insulin secretion, or both. Up to 21 million Americans have diabetes; of those, most have type 2 diabetes (>90%). As many as 4 to 6 million Americans have this metabolic disorder but have not currently been diagnosed. The prevalence is especially high in black and Hispanic persons.

It is predicted that the number of diabetics will increase to 30.3 million Americans and to 366 million people worldwide by 2030 (**Figure 2.1**). Diabetes is more prevalent with increasing age, affecting 8.7% of people aged 20 years and older (**Figure 2.2**), but 17.7% of those ≥60 years of age. This increase in the prevalence of diabetes is primarily due to changing population demographics, including:
- Increasing obesity
- Sedentary lifestyle
- An aging population with a growing percentage of minority populations with a disproportionately high prevalence of diabetes (in the United States) (**Figure 2.3**).

The chronic hyperglycemia of diabetes is associated with long-term vascular damage or dysfunction and the failure of various organs, especially the heart, brain, kidneys, eyes, and nerves (**Figure 2.4**). Diabetes markedly decreases the life span of both men and women (**Figure 2.5**). Health care costs to treat complications related to diabetes exceed $300 billion an-

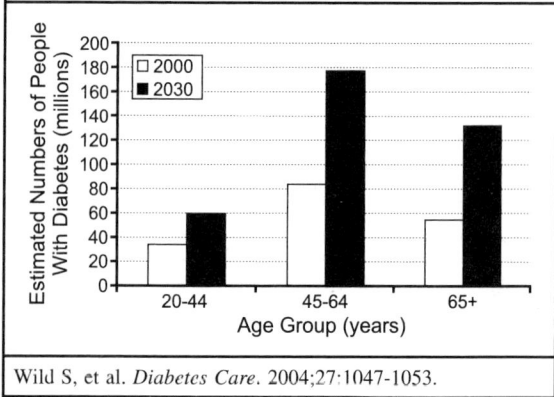

FIGURE 2.1 — Estimated Number of Adults Worldwide With Diabetes by Age Group and Year

Wild S, et al. *Diabetes Care*. 2004;27:1047-1053.

nually. Diabetes-related complications will increasingly consume a disproportionate share of health care resources unless vigorous efforts are made to control them.

Development of Diabetes

It is clear that our aging population, our increasing minority population (especially Hispanics), and the increase in obesity now seen in a high percentage of children will result in striking increases in the prevalence of type 2 diabetes in the United States over the next decade. The current epidemic of obesity (**Figure 2.6**) is probably the single biggest factor in the great increase in type 2 diabetes that is occurring worldwide (**Figure 2.1**).

Several pathophysiologic abnormalities are involved in the development of diabetes. These vary from autoimmune destruction of the β-cells of the pancreas (type 1 diabetes) with consequent insulin deficiency to abnormalities that result in resistance to the

FIGURE 2.2 — Prevalence of Diabetes Among People ≥20 Years of Age: United States, 2002

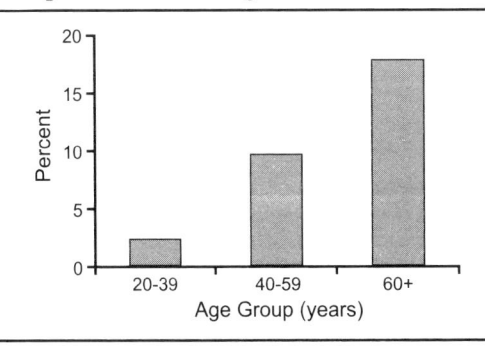

This graph shows the percentage of US adults aged ≥20 years who had diabetes in the year 2002. The percentage of adults with diabetes was 2.2% among those aged 20-39 years, 9.5% aged 40-59 years, and 17.7% aged ≥60 years.

Centers for Disease Control and Prevention (CDC), National diabetes fact sheet: general information and national estimates for diabetes in the United States, 2002. Atlanta, Ga: US Department of Health and Human Services, Centers for Disease Control and Prevention, 2003.

actions of insulin (type 2). The majority of cases of diabetes fall into two broad pathogenetic categories. In one category (type 1 diabetes), the cause is an absolute deficiency of insulin secretion. Persons at increased risk for developing this type of diabetes can often be identified by serologic evidence of an autoimmune pathologic process occurring in the pancreatic islets and by genetic markers. Most often, however, patients are identified when symptoms occur, such as polyuria, thirst, weight loss, dryness and itching of the skin, etc. In the much more prevalent category (type 2 diabetes), the cause is usually a combination of resistance to insulin action and an inadequate compensatory β-cell insulin secretory response. In the latter

FIGURE 2.3 — Age-Specific Prevalence of Diagnosed Diabetes by Race/Ethnicity and Gender: United States, 2002

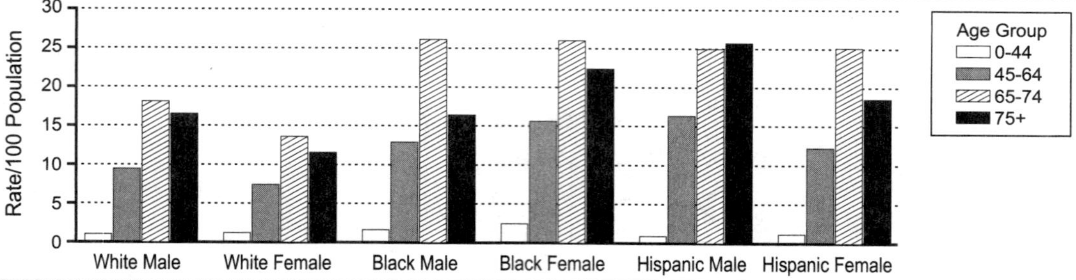

The prevalence of diagnosed diabetes is higher for blacks and Hispanics than for whites across all age groups. Regardless of race-ethnicity and gender, prevalence tended to be highest among persons aged 65-74 and lowest among persons <45 years of age.

Centers for Disease Control and Prevention (CDC), National Center for Health Statistics, Division of Health Interview Statistics, data from the National Health Interview Survey. US Bureau of the Census, census of the population and population estimates. Data computed by the CDC's division of Diabetes Translation, National Center for Chronic Disease Prevention and Health Promotion.

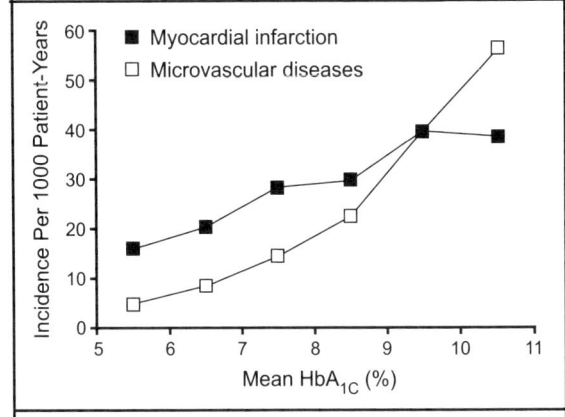

FIGURE 2.4 — United Kingdom Prospective Diabetic Study: Epidemiology

Abbreviation: HbA$_{1C}$, glycosylated hemoglobin

Incidence of both myocardial infarction and microvascular diseases (proteinuria and retinopathy) increases as HbA$_{1C}$ increases. New definitions indicate that a level above 7% requires aggressive therapy.

Stratton IM, et al. *BMJ*. 2000;321:405-412.

category (>90% of diabetics in the United States), subtle hyperglycemia sufficient to cause pathologic and functional changes in target tissues, but without clinical symptoms, may exist for a long period of time before clinical diabetes is diagnosed. In other words, such patients may actually secrete an excess amount of insulin for many years but peripheral utilization is decreased, ie, there is increased insulin resistance and blood glucose levels will be at high normal (up to 126 mg/dL fasting). Eventually, the pancreas is unable to keep up with the demand for extra insulin. During this asymptomatic period, it is often possible to demonstrate an abnormality in carbohydrate metabolism by finding elevated plasma glucose or insulin levels following an oral glucose load. This functional abnormal-

FIGURE 2.5 — Diabetes Reduces Years of Life

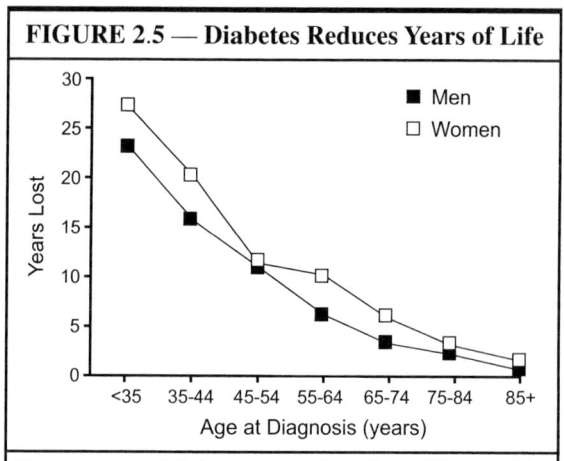

The presence of diabetes markedly reduces life span. For example, a 45- to 54-year old man or woman diagnosed as a diabetic has a life expectancy 10 years less than a nondiabetic (this may have changed recently with more effective therapy for diabetes and comorbid conditions).

Morgan CL, et al. *Diabetes Care.* 2000;23:1103.

ity of impaired glucose tolerance is often a precursor to clinical type 2 diabetes.

Close to 10% of Americans have impaired glucose tolerance and are at risk for the development of clinical diabetes. Risk factors for progression from impaired glucose tolerance include:
- Obesity (**Table 2.1** and **Figure 2.6**)
- Hypertension
- Limited physical activity
- Certain medications (ie, steroids)
- Aging.

There is also a genetic component to diabetes; the development of the disease is more common when there are close relatives with diabetes and in certain minority populations such as blacks, Native Americans, and

FIGURE 2.6 — Increase in Prevalence of Obesity Over the Past Decade (%)

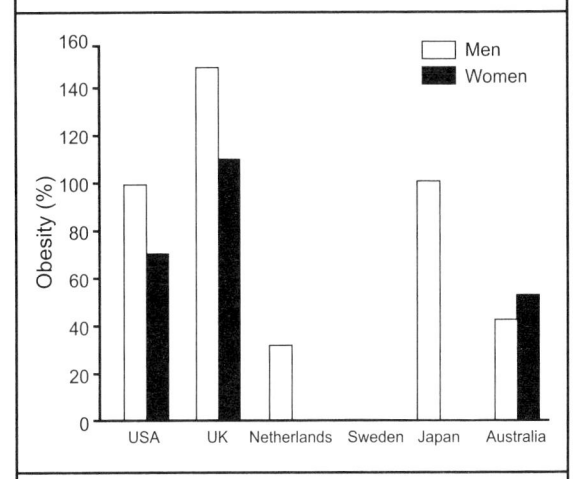

Obesity (defined as ≥20% above ideal weight) has dramatically increased over the past 10 years, not only in the United States, but worldwide.

Sorensen TI. *Diabetes Care*. 2000;23(suppl 2):B1.

Hispanics. However, it appears that socioeconomic factors, including diet and inactivity, play a role in the higher prevalence of diabetes in these minority populations. People displaying a clinical syndrome of central or abdominal obesity (waist measurement >40 inches in men and >34 inches in women), hypertension, insulin resistance/impaired glucose tolerance, hypercoagulability, microalbuminuria, and dyslipidemia have an increased likelihood of developing clinical diabetes. Suggested criteria for testing populations who are at high risk for clinical diabetes are shown in **Table 2.2**.

Type 2 diabetes is frequently not diagnosed until complications appear and many of these patients will have underlying cardiovascular disease at the time of diabetes diagnosis. Although the diagnosis of type 2

TABLE 2.1 — Metabolic and Cardiovascular Risk Factors Associated With Visceral Obesity

- Insulin resistance
- Hyperinsulinemia
- Low high-density lipoprotein cholesterol
- High triglyceride concentrations
- Increased Apo B concentrations
- Increased fibrinogen concentrations
- Increased plasminogen activator
- Increased inhibitor C-reactive protein
- Increased systolic and diastolic blood pressure (BP)
- Increased blood viscosity
- Increased left ventricular muscle mass
- Premature atherosclerosis (coronary heart disease and stroke)
- Microalbuminuria
- Loss of nocturnal reductions in BP and heart rates.

diabetes increases with advancing age, the diagnosis is increasingly being made in younger persons, including children and adolescents. The increasing rates of type 2 diabetes in children and adults parallel the increase in overweight (body mass index [BMI] of 25 to 30 kg/m^2) and obesity (BMI >30 kg/m^2) in the United States. Several recently published lifestyle prevention studies have demonstrated the effectiveness of lifestyle modifications, namely, diet and exercise, in the prevention of type 2 diabetes. There is also evidence that angiotensin-converting enzyme (ACE) inhibitors, angiotensin II receptor blockers (ARBs), metformin, thiazolidinediones, and the α-glucosidase inhibitor acarbose can decrease or slow the rate of the development of type 2 diabetes in predisposed persons.

TABLE 2.2 — Criteria for Testing for Diabetes in Asymptomatic, Undiagnosed Individuals

- Testing for diabetes should be considered in all individuals >45 years of age and if blood glucose levels are normal (ie, <126 mg/dL), it should be repeated at 3-year intervals
- Testing should be considered at a younger age or be carried out more frequently in individuals who:
  - Are obese ($\geq$120% desirable body weight or a body mass index $\geq$27 kg/m^2)
  - Have a first-degree relative with diabetes
  - Are members of a high-risk ethnic population (eg, blacks, Hispanics, Native Americans)
  - Have delivered an infant weighing >9 lb or have been diagnosed with gestational diabetes mellitus
  - Are hypertensive (blood pressure $\geq$140/90 mm Hg)
  - Have a high-density lipoprotein cholesterol level $\leq$35 mg/dL and/or a triglyceride level $\geq$250 mg/dL
  - On previous testing, had impaired glucose tolerance or an elevated fasting glucose level (>126 mg/dL).

Diagnostic Criteria for Diabetes

The diagnosis of diabetes mellitus can be made in three ways as shown in **Table 2.3**, and each should be confirmed at another time by any one of these three methods. The first would include symptoms of diabetes, plus a casual (nonfasting) plasma glucose concentration $\geq$200 mg/dL. A second would be that of a fasting glucose $\geq$126 mg/dL, and the third diagnostic criterion would be a 2-hour postprandial or postglucose load of $\geq$200 mg/dL. Accordingly, the presence of symptoms with a casual plasma glucose of $\geq$200 mg/dL, confirmed on another day by a fasting plasma glucose $\geq$126 mg/dL or a 2-hour postload glucose $\geq$200 mg/dL, would confirm a diagnosis of clinical diabetes.

Undiagnosed type 2 diabetes is common in the United States, with recent estimates that as many as 5

TABLE 2.3 — Criteria for the Diagnosis of Diabetes Mellitus

One or more of the following must be present:

- Symptoms of diabetes plus casual plasma glucose concentration ≥200 mg/dL (11.1 mmol/L). Casual is defined as any time of day without regard to time since last meal. The classic symptoms of diabetes include:
  - Polyuria
  - Polydipsia
  - Unexplained weight loss
- Fasting plasma glucose ≥126 mg/dL (7.0 mmol/L). Fasting is defined as no caloric intake for at least 8 hours
- Two-hour postload glucose ≥200 mg/dL (11.1 mmol/L) during an oral glucose tolerance test (OGTT). The test should be performed as described by the World Health Organization, using a glucose load containing the equivalent of 75-g anhydrous glucose dissolved in water

In the absence of unequivocal hyperglycemia, these criteria should be confirmed by repeat testing on a different day. The third measure (OGTT) is not recommended for routine clinical use.

American Diabetes Association. *Diabetes Care*. 2004;27(suppl 1):S5-S10.

million persons with this disease are currently undiagnosed. Relevant to this issue is the epidemiologic evidence that diabetic retinopathy (most common cause of new blindness in the United States) begins to develop at least 7 years before the clinical diagnosis of type 2 diabetes is made. Patients with undiagnosed diabetes are also at significantly greater risk for ischemic heart disease, stroke, peripheral vascular disease, and diabetic renal disease. Thus it is important to recognize factors that suggest a high risk for diabetes so appropriate screening and treatment can be carried out.

A relationship that has been recently appreciated is the increased prevalence of type 2 diabetes among persons with hepatitis C virus (HCV) infection in the United States. This relationship is especially strong in persons >40 years of age, nonwhites, those with a high BMI, and individuals of lower socioeconomic status. For example, persons ≥40 years of age with HCV infection are more than three times as likely to have type 2 diabetes as those without HCV infection. Since approximately 2.7 million persons in the United States have chronic HCV infections, this represents another high-risk group that should be screened for type 2 diabetes.

Pathogenesis of Type 2 Diabetes

Two major pathophysiologic factors contribute to the development of type 2 diabetes:
- Insulin resistance
- Impaired pancreatic β-cell function.

■ Insulin Resistance

Insulin resistance is relatively common in adults in the United States. Data from the Insulin Resistance Atherosclerosis Study show that 90% of obese African Americans, Caucasians, and Hispanic Americans with type 2 diabetes may be classified as insulin insensitive or resistant. Insulin resistance in conjunction with hyperinsulinemia has also been identified more than a decade before the onset of diabetes in the obese offspring of persons with type 2 diabetes.

Insulin resistance is associated with diminished glucose disposal and dyslipidemia. In skeletal muscle, the major tissue involved in glucose disposal, there is deficient insulin-mediated glucose transport with subsequent impairment of oxidation and glycogen storage. In the liver, insulin resistance is associated with reduced postprandial glucose storage and the ability of insulin to inhibit lipolysis to suppress glycogenolysis and gluconeogenesis in the fasting and postprandial states. The ability of insulin to inhibit lipolysis in adipose tissue is also diminished.

Insulin resistance is associated with a litany of metabolic and hemodynamic abnormalities known as the cardiometabolic syndrome.

Studies in high-risk populations suggest that the insulin-resistant phenotype, like type 2 diabetes, has a genetic component. To date, however, no genetic defect has been found in the majority of patients with type 2 diabetes that would explain their metabolic disease solely due to insulin resistance. Environmental factors appear to be the main determinant of insulin resistance.

■ Impaired Pancreatic β-Cell Function

Most patients who are obese and insulin resistant do not develop diabetes. They have the ability to compensate for insulin resistance by increasing their insulin secretion. Therefore, the development of type 2 diabetes involves a defect in compensatory insulin secretion.

Possible causes of β-cell dysfunction, the other major causative factor in diabetes, include:
- Amyloid deposition or inflammation/apoptosis or other conditions that reduce β-cell mass
- Sustained insulin resistance leading to β-cell exhaustion
- Glucose and/or lipid toxicity to β-cells
- Autoimmune β-cell destruction.

According to data from the United Kingdom Prospective Diabetes Study, β-cell function was reduced 50% at the time of diagnosis of type 2 diabetes, and there was progressive loss of function over time.

SELECTED READING

American Diabetes Association. Standards of medical care for patients with diabetes mellitus. *Diabetes Care*. 2004;27(suppl 1):S15-S35.

Boyle JP, Honeycutt AA, Narayan KM, et al. Projection of diabetes burden through 2050: impact of changing demography and disease prevalence in the U.S. *Diabetes Care*. 2001;24:1936-1940.

Buchanan TA, Xiang AH, Peters RK, et al. Preservation of pancreative beta-cell function and prevention of type 2 diabetes by pharmacological treatment of insulin resistance in high-risk Hispanic women. *Diabetes*. 2002;51:2796-2803.

Chiasson JL, Josse RG, Gomis R, Hanefeld M, Karasik A, Laakso M; STOP-NIDDM Trial Research Group. Acarbose for prevention of type 2 diabetes mellitus: the STOP-NIDDM randomised trial. *Lancet*. 2002;359:2072-2077.

Edelman SV, Henry RR. *Diagnosis and Management of Type 2 Diabetes*. 5th ed. Caddo, Okla: Professional Communications, Inc; 2002.

Gerich JE. Contibutions of insulin-resistance and insulin-secretory defects to the pathogenesis of type 2 diabetes mellitus. *Mayo Clin Proc*. 2003;78:447-456.

Knowler WC, Barrett-Connor E, Fowler SE, et al; Diabetes Prevention Program Research Group. Reduction in the incidence of type 2 diabetes with lifestyle intervention or metformin. *N Engl J Med*. 2002;346:393-403.

Mehta SH, Brancati FL, Sulkowski MS, Strathdee SA, Szklo M, Thomas DL. Prevalence of type 2 diabetes mellitus among persons with hepatitis C virus infection in the United States. *Ann Intern Med*. 2000;133:592-599.

Mokdad AH, Ford ES, Bowman BA, et al. Prevalence of obesity, diabetes, and obesity-related health risk factors, 2001. *JAMA*. 2003;289:76-79.

Sowers JR, Haffner S. Treatment of cardiovascular and renal risk factors in the diabetic hypertensive. *Hypertension*. 2002;40:781-788.

Sowers JR, Lester MA. Diabetes and cardiovascular disease. *Diabetes Care*. 1999;22(suppl 3):C14-C20.

Stratton IM, Adler A, Neil HA, et al. Association of glycaemia with macrovascular and microvascular complications of type 2 diabetes (UKPDS 35): prospective observational study. *BMJ*. 2000;321:405-412.

Tuomilehto J, Lindstrom J, Eriksson JG, et al; Finnish Diabetes Prevention Study Group. Prevention of type 2 mellitus by changes in lifestyle among subjects with impaired glucose tolerance. *N Engl J Med*. 2001;344:1343-1350.

3

Scope of and Risk Factors for Cardiovascular Disease in Diabetic Patients

Cardiovascular Disease in Diabetics

Whereas cardiovascular disease (CVD) accounts for 40% of the overall mortality in the United States, nearly 80% of deaths in type 2 diabetic persons are secondary to complications of CVD, such as:
- Sudden death
- Myocardial infarction (MI)
- Congestive heart failure (CHF)
- Cerebrovascular and peripheral vascular disease.

All of the above complications are considerably more common in diabetics than in nondiabetics. The risk for CVD mortality is approximately 2-fold in diabetic men and 4-fold in diabetic women when compared with people without diabetes. The relative risk for stroke in persons with diabetes is 2- to 3-fold higher than in nondiabetic persons and is higher in females than in males. The United Kingdom Prospective Diabetes Study (UKPDS) group found that over an 8-year period, increased risk for stroke in diabetic persons was related to a diagnosis of hypertension or to higher systolic blood pressure (SBP), regardless of whether the blood pressure (BP) was measured in treated or untreated persons. Even people with SBP between 125 and 142 mm Hg had twice the risk for stroke observed in persons with lower levels of SBP. Information from death certificates indicates that hypertension is implicated in many of the deaths coded to diabetes and that diabetes is involved in over 10% of deaths coded to hypertension-related disease. While much of the attention relating to diabetes treatment has centered on prevention of diabetic nephropathy and end-stage renal disease (ESRD), CVD is far more common as an outcome in this population.

It is important to emphasize that some, but not all, recent data suggest that a diabetic without a history of myocardial infarction (MI) is at the same risk for a cardiovascular (CV) event as a nondiabetic patient with a history of an MI (**Figure 3.1**). In other words, any diabetic patient should be considered at high risk for CVD. This reconsideration is important in therapy considerations (see Chapter 4, *Pathophysiologic/Metabolic Interactions Between Diabetes and Cardiovascular Disease*, and Chapter 5, *The Renin-Angiotensin-Aldosterone System in Diabetes*).

■ Microvascular Disease in Diabetes
Diabetic Retinopathy

Certain complications are specific to the diabetic patient. Diabetic retinopathy is the most common cause of new blindness in Americans between the ages of 20 and 74 in the United States. In patients with type 2 diabetes, early manifestations of retinopathy (typically microaneurysm) noted as dot or punctate hemorrhages are common within 5 years after diagnosis of diabetes. Up to 90% of these patients will have some evidence of retinopathy by 15 years postdiagnosis. The presence of proliferative retinopathy is progressive over the course of both type 1 and type 2 diabetes.

Type 1 diabetics should be evaluated by an ophthalmologist yearly, starting 5 years after diagnosis of diabetes. Type 2 diabetic patients should have an ophthalmologic evaluation yearly, starting from the time of diagnosis. Because of accelerated disease during pregnancy, ophthalmologic evaluation is recommended

FIGURE 3.1 — Risk of Cardiovascular Events in Type 2 Diabetes

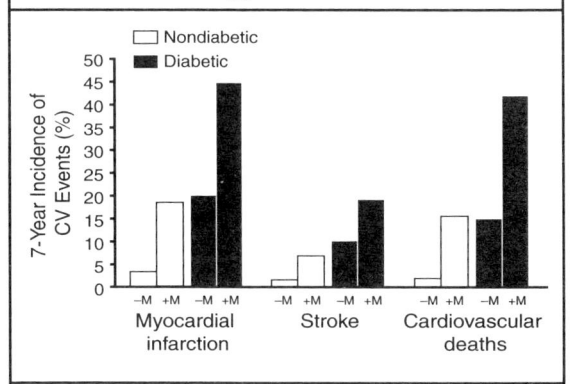

Key: –M, no prior MI; +M, prior MI.

Type 2 diabetes is associated with a marked increase in the risk of cardiovascular (CV) disease. Seven-year incidences of fatal or nonfatal myocardial infarction (MI), fatal or nonfatal stroke, and death from CV causes among 1373 nondiabetic subjects were compared with the incidences among 1059 patients with type 2 diabetes. Both the presence of diabetes and the history of a previous MI at baseline were associated with an increased incidence of CV events. In both diabetic patients and nondiabetic subjects, history of prior MI at baseline was significantly associated with an increased incidence of MI, stroke, and CV death. Diabetic patients without prior MI, however, had as high a CV risk as nondiabetic subjects with previous MI.

Haffner SM, et al. *N Engl J Med.* 1998;339:229-234.

during the first trimester, with follow-up throughout pregnancy.

Treatment of diabetic retinopathy primarily involves laser photocoagulation. Focal coagulation is done for the destruction of new vessels or treatment of clinically significant macular edema. Panretinal photocoagulation (sparing the macula) is conducted to destroy ischemic retina and decrease the stimulus to neovascularization. The intent of such therapy is to regress neovascularization and decrease the risk of subsequent hemorrhage. This technique, however, can exacerbate preexisting macular edema, especially if applied too aggressively.

Diabetic Neuropathy

Diabetic neuropathy is another specific complication of diabetes. This is most commonly manifested by orthostatic hypotension.

Diabetic Nephropathy

Approximately 30% to 35% of persons with type 1 diabetes will develop nephropathy. The likelihood of type 2 patients developing nephropathy is less, but because of the 10-fold greater prevalence of type 2 diabetes, it is the leading cause of ESRD.

The first laboratory abnormality that indicates the development of diabetic nephropathy is the appearance of small quantities of albumin in the urine, microalbuminuria, sometimes referred to as "incipient diabetic nephropathy" (**Table 3.1**). When the level of albumin is measurable by conventional dipstick, it is referred

TABLE 3.1 — Definitions of Abnormalities in Albumin Excretion*

Category	24-h Collection	Spot Collection
Normal	<30 mg/24 h	<30 µg/min creatinine
Microalbuminuria	30-300 mg/24 h	30-300 µg/min creatinine
Clinical albuminuria	>300 mg/24 h	>300 µg/min creatinine

* Screen for albuminuria once a year (dipstick); if negative, check for microalbuminuria (Micral test)

to as clinical albuminuria. This indicates a progressive fall in the glomerular filtration rate (GFR). The rate of progression from microalbuminuria to clinical albuminuria and the rate of decline in GFR are both modifiable by treatment (see Chapter 4, *Pathophysiologic/Metabolic Interactions Between Diabetes and Cardiovascular Disease*).

General Treatment Strategies if Microalbuminuria is Detected

Several guidelines committees have recommended rigorous glycemic control to decrease the likelihood of the development of microalbuminuria and to delay the progression of microalbuminuria in both type 1 and type 2 patients with preexisting microalbuminuria.

Early studies from the STENO diabetes center in Denmark showed that even modest control of hypertension with triple-drug therapy (diuretic/β-blocker/vasodilator) could strikingly decrease the decline of GFR in patient with established diabetic nephropathy. These studies established the importance of rigorous BP control, presaging the current recommendations of a treatment goal of <130/80 mm Hg in diabetic patients. The unique role of angiotensin-converting enzyme (ACE) inhibitors and angiotensin II receptor blockers (ARBs) as part of this treatment strategy is discussed in Chapter 7, *Cardiovascular Risk Reduction in Hypertensive Diabetics*.

Cardiovascular Disease in Diabetic Women

The incidence of CVD increases with increasing age in the United States and other westernized countries, and elderly women constitute a disproportionate component of the aging population. In the United States each year, >240,000 women die from MI and

>88,000 die from stroke. For a 50-year-old woman, the lifetime risk of having coronary heart disease (CHD) is 46% and the risk of dying from this disease is 32%. Despite a decrease in CHD mortality in most developed countries, the absolute number of CHD deaths in the elderly, particularly in aging diabetic women, has increased substantially.

Population demographics suggest that in the United States, the number of persons >80 years of age in 25 to 30 years will increase dramatically. The number of women in this age group is and will continue to be disproportionately high.

Although CVD is generally less prevalent in premenopausal women than in age-matched men, this difference disappears after menopause, presumably related to decreased estrogen production. In diabetes (type 1 *or* type 2), this gender difference in CVD is not seen in people <50 years of age, probably because the metabolic and hemodynamic benefits of endogenous estradiol are canceled by the diabetic syndrome. Recent controlled clinical trials underscore the critical importance of aggressively treating CVD risk factors, especially dyslipidemia and hypertension, in women with diabetes. However, hormone replacement therapy (HRT) is not generally indicated for these postmenopausal women given their marked propensity for hypercoagulability, suggesting a possible increase in CVD risk with HRT.

Cardiovascular disease, not ESRD, is the leading cause of death in women with diabetes (as it is in men). In the Framingham Study, MI, angina, and sudden death were 2-fold higher in diabetic than in nondiabetic persons. In addition to removing the normal premenopausal CVD protection, diabetes is a greater CVD mortality risk factor in women than in men >50 years of age. Women with diabetes are also more likely to die after an MI than nondiabetic women or men with or without diabetes. The risk of death from CHD in women with diabetes is >3-fold that in nondiabetic women.

Many factors contribute to the increase in CVD in diabetic women as well as in men, including:
- Hypertension
- Lipoprotein abnormalities
- Endothelial dysfunction
- Increased vascular oxidative stress
- Reduced vascular compliance
- Enhanced platelet aggregation/adhesion
- Enhanced coagulation/reduced fibrinolysis.

Risk Factors

Diabetes itself should be considered an independent risk factor for CVD in men and women. Other major risk factors for CVD in diabetics as well as in other individuals include:
- Smoking
- Elevated BP
- Abnormal serum lipids and lipoproteins.

But in diabetes, hyperglycemia and insulin resistance increase the significance of these risk factors. Other predisposing risk factors for the development of CVD in patients with diabetes include:
- Obesity
- Physical inactivity
- Family history of CVD
- Advancing age.

These are similar to the risk factors contributing to insulin resistance.

The metabolic syndrome of insulin resistance, hypertension, abdominal obesity, hyperglycemia, elevated triglycerides, and low levels of high-density lipoprotein cholesterol is now well recognized (Syndrome X). The treatment of the diabetic patient is aimed at correcting as many of the findings in Syndrome X as possible. Several clinical features of the metabolic syndrome are listed in **Table 3.2**.

TABLE 3.2 — Clinical Features of the Metabolic Syndrome*	
Risk Factor	**Criteria for Risk**
Abdominal obesity	
Men	Waist circumference: >38 in
Women	Waist circumference: >34 in
Triglycerides	$\geq$150 mg/dL
HDL cholesterol	
Men	<40 mg/dL
Women	<50 mg/dL
Blood pressure	$\geq$130/$\geq$85 mm Hg
Impaired glucose tolerance	Serum glucose between 110 and 125 mg/dL
* Defined as consisting of $\geq$3 of the abnormalities listed.	
Abbreviation: HDL, high-density lipoprotein.	

In the Multiple Risk Factor Intervention Trial (MRFIT), >5000 persons with diabetes were observed for 12 years and compared with more than 350,000 without diabetes. The risk of CVD death at 12 years was 3-fold higher in diabetic men compared with controls, regardless of age, ethnicity, cholesterol levels, SBP, or tobacco use. Even when patients had optimal SBP and were nonsmokers, the relative risk of CVD death was still 2.5 times higher in those who were diabetic. The MRFIT study underscored the fact that diabetes is a strong independent risk factor for CVD mortality and that systolic hypertension, hypercholesterolemia, and cigarette smoking are also significant independent predictors of mortality in men with and without diabetes. The presence of one or more of these risk factors, in turn, had a significantly greater bearing on CVD risk in the diabetic than in the nondiabetic cohort. The association of an elevated SBP and CV death in diabetics is especially strong (**Figure 3.2**)

FIGURE 3.2 — Association of Systolic Blood Pressure and Cardiovascular Death in Type 2 Diabetes

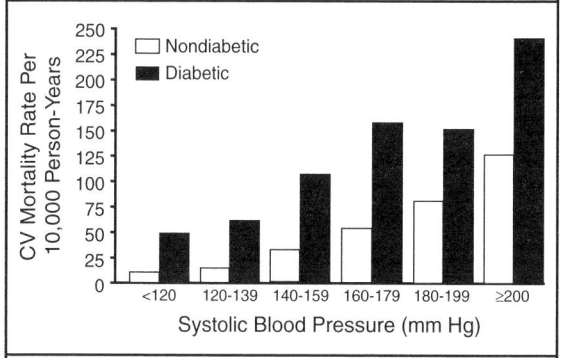

In the Multiple Risk Factor Intervention Trial (MRFIT), the relationships of systolic blood pressure (BP) and other cardiovascular (CV) risk factors to CV mortality were compared in men with diabetes (n = 5163) and without diabetes (n = 342,815). The absolute risk of CV death was 3 times higher for men with diabetes than for those without diabetes. Systolic BP was positively related to the risk of CV death, with a significant trend in both nondiabetic and diabetic subjects (P <0.001). At every level of systolic BP, however, CV death was much greater in men with diabetes than in men without diabetes. The higher the systolic BP, the greater the absolute excess risk for patients with diabetes and the greater potential for prevention of CV death among patients with diabetes by control of elevated BP.

Stamler J, et al. *Diabetes Care*. 1993;16:434-444.

The incidence of both diabetes mellitus and essential hypertension increases with advancing age in industrialized, westernized societies. Data from non-industrialized societies do not demonstrate this striking age-related increase in incidence, underlying the importance of environmental factors such as obesity and a sedentary lifestyle. In industrialized societies, advancing age is often associated with a loss of lean body mass, particularly that of skeletal muscle tissue and bone. Skeletal muscle is the predominant site of insulin action to promote glucose uptake, and the decrease in skeletal muscle tissue likely contributes to the increasing insulin resistance associated with aging. The loss of lean body mass is also associated with an increase in relative body fat, particularly abdominal fat. Abdominal fat, particularly that known as visceral fat located in the mesenteric/omental region, is pathophysiologically linked to insulin resistance, impaired glucose tolerance, and hypertension (see Chapter 4, *Pathophysiologic/Metabolic Interactions Between Diabetes and Cardiovascular Disease*).

Smoking as a Risk Factor

Cigarette smoking is the most important preventable cause of illness and premature death in the United States. There is increasing evidence that cigarette smoking has a synergistic effect with diabetes in raising morbidity and mortality in both type 1 and type 2 diabetic patients. Unfortunately, smoking prevalence among diabetic patients has been reported to be approximately the same as in the general population. Several studies have shown that physician counseling during a simple routine consultation increases the likelihood that patients will stop smoking. A recently reported study indicates that a structured intervention program conducted by a nurse in both primary care and hospital settings can achieve a significant increase in smoking cessation in diabetics. Thus it is imperative that health care providers emphasize the especially high risk attributable to smoking in diabetic patients and the overall health benefits of smoking cessation. Indeed, the high baseline risk for CVD within a 10-year period in diabetics should be emphasized in counseling to promote smoking cessation.

SELECTED READING

American Diabetes Association. Standards of medical care for patients with diabetes mellitus. *Diabetes Care*. 2004;27(suppl 1):S15-S35.

Bell DS. Stroke in the diabetic patient. *Diabetes Care*. 1994;17: 213-219.

Canga N, De Irala J, Vara E, Duaso MJ, Ferrer A, Martinez-Gonzalez MA. Intervention study for smoking cessation in diabetic patients: a randomized controlled trial in both clinical and primary care settings. *Diabetes Care*. 2000;23:1455-1460.

Davis TM, Millns H, Stratton IM, Holman RR, Turner RC. Risk factors for stroke in type 2 diabetes mellitus: United Kingdom Prospective Diabetes Study (UKPDS) 29. *Arch Intern Med*. 1999;159: 1097-1103.

Edelman SV, Henry RR. *Diagnosis and Management of Type 2 Diabetes*. 5th ed. Caddo, Okla: Professional Communications, Inc; 2002.

Haffner SM, Lehto S, Ronnemaa T, Pyorala K, Laakso M. Mortality from coronary heart disease in subjects with type 2 diabetes and in nondiabetic subjects with and without prior myocardial infarction. *N Engl J Med*. 1998;339:229-234.

Haire-Joshu D, Glasgow RE, Tibbs TL. Smoking and diabetes. *Diabetes Care*. 1999;22:1887-1898.

Hypertension in Diabetes Study Group. Hypertension in Diabetes Study (HDS):1. Prevalence of hypertension in newly presenting type 2 diabetic patients and the association with risk factors for cardiovascular and diabetic complications. *J Hypertens*. 1993;11: 309-317.

Report of the Expert Committee on Diagnosis and Classification of Diabetes Mellitus. *Diabetes Care*. 1997;20:1183-1197.

Sowers JR, Epstein M, Frohlich ED. Diabetes, hypertension, and cardiovascular disease: an update. *Hypertension*. 2001;37:1053-1059.

Stratton IM, Adler A, Neil HA, et al. Association of glycaemia with macrovascular and microvascular complications of type 2 diabetes (UKPDS 35): prospective observational study. *BMJ*. 2000; 321:405-412.

4

Pathophysiologic/Metabolic Interactions Between Diabetes and Cardiovascular Disease

Obesity, Insulin Resistance, and Hypertension

The relationship between visceral adiposity, mesenteric and omental fat, and insulin resistance has been extensively investigated. It has been found that insulin resistance is closely related to visceral or abdominal obesity. Interventions designed to prevent the accumulation of visceral fat (ie, caloric restriction and exercise) have been shown to decrease age-related increases in insulin resistance and impaired glucose tolerance. Based on this and other experimental data, it appears that insulin resistance associated with visceral adiposity is caused, in part, by abnormalities in fatty acid metabolism. This notion is grounded in the observation that both mesenteric and omental fat are resistant to the actions of insulin. This results in accelerated lipolysis or breakdown of fatty material. The increased release of free fatty acids (FFAs) into the portal blood supply, in turn, lends to hepatic overproduction of triglycerides and a decrease in the synthesis of high-density lipoprotein (HDL) (characteristic abnormalities seen in both diabetes and hypertension) (**Table 2.1**).

In addition, increased fatty acids tend to increase skeletal muscle resistance to the actions of insulin. This, in turn, leads to a reduced metabolism of triglyceride-rich particles like very low-density lipoprotein (VLDL). Triglycerides are also increased by this mechanism and HDL levels are decreased.

Increased FFA also contributes to impaired vascular endothelial-derived vasodilation. Thus increased FFA represents one of the important links between obesity, insulin resistance, and the development of hypertension, an integral component of the cardiometabolic syndrome in blood pressure (BP) ≥130/85 mm Hg.

The age-related increase in fat mass is greater in women than in men. There is an acceleration in central adipose tissue that occurs postmenopausally. This increase in visceral adiposity may account for increases in the prevalence of hypertension and diabetes in postmenopausal women. Regularly performed exercise may protect against, but does not abolish, the increase in "fatness" with aging. One investigation showed that even when master athletes maintain optimal exercise intensity and duration, body fat still increased by approximately 27% in those >65 years of age over a 10-year period. Physically active men and women have less central adiposity than their sedentary counterparts. Exercise intervention studies have shown that endurance training selectively reduces body fat centrally. These observations are important in that visceral adiposity is strongly associated with diabetes, hypertension, and cardiovascular disease (CVD).

Population-based surveys of adults have revealed that as many as 50% of persons with hypertension have glucose intolerance. The majority of hypertensive persons demonstrating this characteristic are obese. Studies have also demonstrated, however, that even hypertensive persons with normal weight may have impaired glucose metabolism. Data have repeatedly confirmed that reduced insulin sensitivity is not uncommon even in lean persons with hypertension, ie, more insulin is required to handle a glucose load in insulin-resistant than in insulin-sensitive persons. It has been suggested that the insulin resistance and impaired glucose tolerance associated with essential hypertension may be due to decreased skeletal muscle blood flow as a result of vasoconstriction or a deficit in insulin-receptor pathways.

Persons with hypertension display other metabolic abnormalities that are also generally seen in diabetes. As noted, they generally have lower levels of HDL, higher levels of triglycerides and VLDL, and abnormal small, dense, and more atherogenic low-density lipoprotein (LDL) particles (**Table 4.1**) when compared with normotensive individuals of the same age and weight. In addition, factors such as increase in the fibrinogen that enhance the tendency for clotting are increased and fibrinolytic activity is decreased; hence the need for therapy (aspirin) designed to decrease clotting tendencies to reduce risk of CVD.

TABLE 4.1 — Lipoprotein Abnormalities in Patients With Hypertension as Well as in Those With Diabetes Mellitus

- Increased plasma levels of:
  - VLDL
  - LDL
  - Lipoprotein (a)
- Decreased plasma HDL cholesterol
- Increased plasma triglyceride levels
- Increased lipoprotein oxidation
- Increased small dense LDL cholesterol products
- Decreased lipoprotein lipase activity

Abbreviations: HDL, high-density lipoprotein; LDL, low-density lipoprotein; VLDL, very low-density lipoprotein.

Genetic studies, including parent-child, twin, and gene studies have yielded data suggesting a genetic basis for the relationship between hypertension and the metabolic abnormalities noted in diabetes. For example, there are higher heritability tendencies in twins compared with nontwin siblings for BP, LDL, VLDL, and body mass index (BMI) changes. Almost 70% of adults with hypertension before age 55 years have siblings or parents with hypertension, and 12% of all hypertensive persons have dyslipidemia as well as hypertension. Thus both hypertension and diabetes have a genetic basis, and both conditions have been linked to insulin resistance. It is not a given, however, that if there is diabetes with hypertension in the family, offspring will necessarily inherit these conditions.

Hypertension and Diabetes

As noted, persons with essential or primary hypertension manifest insulin resistance. Persons with hypertension are at least twice as likely as normotensive counterparts to progress to clinical diabetes over a 5-year period. In the early stages of insulin resistance, there is a compensatory increase in insulin secretion and concentration. Over time, pancreatic secretion of insulin may decrease as the pancreas becomes "worn out" and a state of relative deficit of insulin occurs—type 2 diabetes. Insulin normally causes vasodilation in the peripheral vessels. However, when there is insulin resistance as in diabetes and hypertension, there is an impaired vasodilatory response to insulin. Thus insulin resistance may contribute to increased vascular resistance as well as to impaired glucose uptake in insulin-sensitive tissues, such as fat and skeletal muscle.

Recent studies (Captopril Prevention Project [CAPPP], Heart Outcomes Prevention Evaluation [HOPE], Valsartan Antihypertensive Long-term Use Evaluation [VALUE], and Antihypertensive and Lipid-Lowering Treatment to Prevent Heart Attack Trial [ALLHAT]) indicate that angiotensin II interferes with insulin action in vascular tissues, perhaps explaining the recent observations that angiotensin-converting enzyme (ACE) inhibition or the use of an angiotensin II receptor blocker (ARB) decreases the chances of hypertensive patients progressing to type 2 diabetes compared with regimens that do not include these agents. Insulin resistance in patients with hypertension may also be related to alterations in blood flow to skeletal muscle (**Figure 4.1**). In hypertensive states, there is hypertrophy and constriction of the small nutrient vessels that collectively may contribute to decreased delivery of insulin and glucose to skeletal muscle. Thus there is a need for more insulin to metabolize glucose that is present (ie, diminished insulin sensitivity). Also, in hypertensive persons, particularly those who are sedentary, there may be a preponderance of insulin-resistant type II muscle fibers. In contrast, active normotensive persons have relatively more type I skeletal muscle fibers that are insulin sensitive. Thus agents that increase nutrient delivery to skeletal muscle tissues (ie, ACE inhibitors) or other vasodilators (through effects on small vessels) and exercise (through increasing insulin-sensitive red muscle fibers) could diminish the chances of hypertensive individuals developing diabetes (**Figure 4.2**). An ACE inhibitor or an ARB may also correct some of the angiotensin II–induced insulin-signaling pathway abnormalities that contribute to insulin resistance in hypertensive persons.

Up to 75% of diabetic cardiovascular (CV) and renal complications can be attributed to hypertension, especially systolic hypertension (**Figure 4.3**). High BP also contributes strikingly to the development and the progression of diabetic retinopathy, which, as previously noted, is the leading cause of newly developed blindness in the United States and other industrialized nations.

It is clear that diabetes predisposes a person to hypertension and that hypertension also predisposes people to diabetes. In a recent large prospective study that included 12,550 adults, development of type 2 diabetes was almost 2.5 times as likely in persons with hypertension as in their normotensive counterparts. Es-

FIGURE 4.1 — Pathogenesis of Hypertension in the Insulin-Resistant State

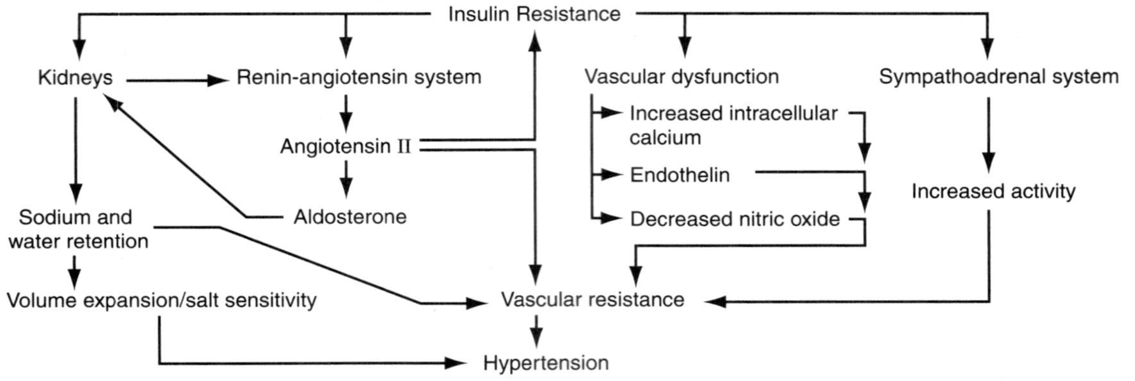

Insulin resistance involves the interaction of abnormalities of the renin-angiotensin-aldosterone system, vascular dysfunction, the sympathetic nervous system, sodium sensitivity, and hypertension. These mechanisms are closely related in the genesis of cardiovascular events.

FIGURE 4.2 — ACE Inhibition

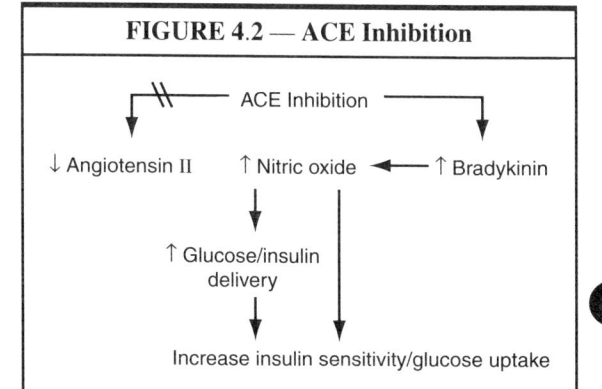

```
            ┌──╫── ACE Inhibition ──┐
            ↓                        ↓
  ↓ Angiotensin II   ↑ Nitric oxide ◄── ↑ Bradykinin
                          ↓
                  ↑ Glucose/insulin
                      delivery
                          ↓
        Increase insulin sensitivity/glucose uptake
```

Angiotensin-converting enzyme (ACE) inhibition increases insulin sensitivity by increasing insulin/glucose delivery to insulin-sensitive tissues. This occurs as a result of a reduction in the generation of angiotensin II, a potent vasoconstrictor that plays a role in decreasing insulin action in peripheral tissues. This effect is also mediated via activation of bradykinin – nitric oxide (a vasodilating substance) and suppression of renin-angiotensin-aldosterone system mechanisms.

sential hypertension accounts for the majority of cases of high BP in persons with type 2 diabetes. Isolated systolic hypertension is also common in diabetics, and supine hypertension with orthostatic hypotension is not uncommon in diabetic persons with autonomic neuropathy.

In summary, insulin resistance or impaired insulin-mediated glucose utilization is an integral component of the cardiometabolic syndrome, which often progresses to type 2 diabetes and CVD events. Hyperinsulinemia, an important component of the cardiometabolic syndrome, may predispose to the development of hypertension, another important part of this syndrome. Hyperinsulinemia may directly contribute to elevated BP by enhancing sympathetic nervous system activity and promoting renal sodium retention. In-

FIGURE 4.3 — Relationship of Elevated Systolic Blood Pressure and Complications of Diabetes

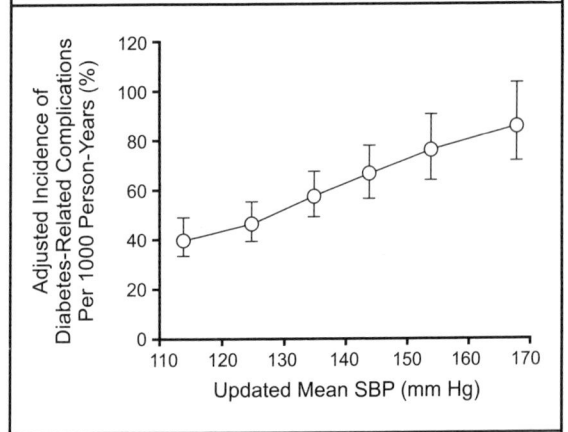

As systolic blood pressure (SBP) rises, diabetic cardiovascular complications increase.

Adler AI, et al. *BMJ*. 2000;321:412-419.

sulin may also indirectly increase BP by decreasing the signaling processes that are important for vascular relaxation. Further, an overexpression of the tissue renin-angiotensin system (RAS) appears to contribute to impaired insulin utilization in skeletal muscle and fat tissue, as well as diminished vasorelaxation. Therapeutic strategies that may improve insulin sensitivity, including those that interrupt the renin-angiotensin-aldosterone system (RAAS), may impede the progression of impaired insulin sensitivity to that of clinical diabetes, as well as reduce BP, renal disease progression, and CVD. This may account for the fact that the occurrence of new-onset diabetes is less in patients treated with an inhibitor of the RAAS.

Circadian Blood Pressure Rhythm in Diabetes

Persons displaying impaired carbohydrate tolerance/insulin resistance as a part of the cardiometabolic syndrome and persons with diabetes often do not have a normal circadian rhythm of BP and heart rate (**Table 4.2**). These persons do not display the normal "dipping" of BP and heart rate that occurs during sleep and are thus termed "nondippers" (**Figure 4.4**). There are other disorders associated with nondipping such as heart failure, autonomic neuropathy, left ventricular hypertrophy (LVH), and sleep disturbances. Nondipping in diabetics may be explained by autonomic neuropathy and impaired baroreflex function. Other factors that may play a role include intravascular volume expansion, cardiac diastolic dysfunction, and enhanced sympathetic/reduced parasympathetic and/or increased RAS activity. One caveat of nondipping is that the daytime determination of BP in such patients may represent an underestimation of the pressure load over 24 hours. Further, elevated nighttime BP has been found to correlate best with microalbuminuria and LVH, which are, in turn, powerful risk predictors for coro-

TABLE 4.2 — Hemodynamic Characteristics of Hypertension in Diabetes

- Increased peripheral vascular resistance
- Enhanced vasoconstrictor responses to vasoagonists
- Decreased vasorelaxation responses, particularly to stimulators of nitric oxide
- Expanded plasma volume
- Supine hypertension with orthostatic hypotension
- Increased incidence of isolated systolic hypertension
- Nondipping of blood pressure at night
- Diminished baroreceptor sensitivity
- Labile hypertension

FIGURE 4.4 — 24-Hour Systolic Blood Pressure Measurements

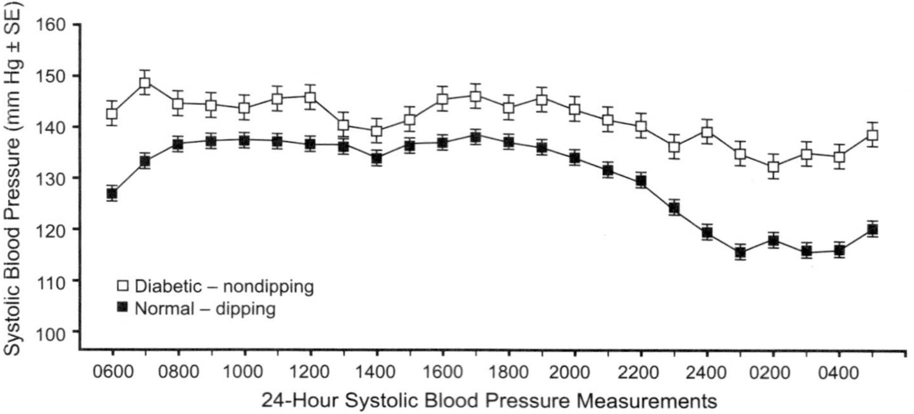

Abbreviation: SE, standard error of measurement.

Diabetic patients frequently do not exhibit the normal decrease of about 10% in blood pressure (BP) during sleep. This "nondipping" status and increased BP during the night may contribute to more vascular injury.

nary heart disease (CHD) and stroke. The nondipping phenomenon provides additional support for more rigorous BP control in diabetics based on daytime BP evaluations.

Hypertension often antedates and appears to contribute to the development of diabetic renal disease. Diabetic nephropathy, which is present after approximately 15 years of diabetes in one third of people with type 1 diabetes and in 20% of those with type 2 diabetes, is an important contributing factor for the development of hypertension in the diabetic individual. High BP associated with diabetic nephropathy is usually characterized by salt and fluid retention and increased peripheral vascular resistance. Indeed, those abnormalities appear to be the hallmarks of hypertension associated with all diabetes.

Increased vascular resistance and enhanced vasoconstricting responses to vasoagonists such as angiotensin II, endothelin, and norepinephrine are found early in the development of hypertension in both type 1 and type 2 diabetes. These enhanced vascular reactivity responses may reflect endothelial dysfunction (ie, decreased availability of a powerful vasodilator, nitric oxide) and small expansions in intravascular volume. Diabetic patients also display reduced baroreceptor sensitivity even prior to overt neuropathy. This reduced baroreflex sensitivity likely contributes to labile hypertension, orthostatic hypotension, and nondipping, all of which are characteristic of the hypertension seen in diabetic patients (**Table 4.2**).

Dyslipidemia and Diabetes

For any lipoprotein level, diabetics have more significant CHD than do those without diabetes, due partly to qualitative differences in the makeup of the lipoproteins. The elevation of triglycerides and the increase in oxidation of lipoproteins that exist in the presence of hyperglycemia are cytotoxic to vascular endothelial cells and help to accelerate atherogenesis. On the other hand, glycation of HDL decreases its half-life through increased clearance. The resulting "diabetogenic" lipid profile consists of elevated triglycerides, reduced HDL, and a very atherogenic oxidized, glycated, small, dense LDL particle.

Because of the atherogenic lipid profile and the fact, as noted previously, that diabetics are at high risk for CVD, it is generally recommended that all diabetic persons undergo a secondary prevention approach, with LDL being lowered to <100 mg/dL, HDL increased to >45 mg/dL, and triglycerides decreased to <200 mg/dL if at all possible—just as if they already had experienced a vascular event. Recent data suggest that in these high-risk patients, an LDL target of <70 mg/dL leads to a better outcome than a target level of <100 mg/dL.

Endothelial Dysfunction

Recognition of the importance of the vascular endothelium in maintaining vascular health has evolved over the past decade. Nitric oxide (NO), a potent vasodilator derived from vascular endothelial and smooth muscle cells, is an important modulator of local vascular tone, platelet aggregation and adhesion, and thrombus formation. Abnormal vascular NO metabolism has been observed in diabetes, hypertension, dyslipidemia, unstable angina, and congestive heart failure. These abnormalities may occur due to decreased production and/or increased destruction of NO produced by the vasculature. Increased destruction of NO can occur with oxidative destruction of the NO molecule. Superoxide anions generated by oxidative stress interact with NO, reducing its functional properties and promoting the formation of substances that cause cellular damage. Oxidative stress is a result of the excess generation of toxic oxygen free radicals which may occur with smoking or excessive activity of the RAAS. Overexpression of the RAAS as exists in CV tissues in the diabetic state contributes to the increased production of these toxic products. Inhibition of the ACE and the decreased conversion of angiotensin I to angiotensin II has been shown to improve endothelial function in patients with coronary artery disease and associated CVD risks. This may partially explain the benefits of ACE inhibition in several recent trials in patients with CVD over and above their effect on BP.

Hyperglycemia, hypertension, and dyslipidemia act cumulatively to cause endothelial dysfunction (**Table 4.3**). Hyperglycemia causes enhanced destruction of NO. It has also been reported that high glucose levels, independent of osmolar effects, attenuate cytokine-induced stimulation of NO production by vascular smooth muscle cells. Hyperglycemia, hypertension, and dyslipidemia may all contribute to endothelial dysfunction. With endothelial dysfunction, there is increased endothelial adhesion of monocytes, platelets, and neutrophils; an accelerated disappearance of

---

TABLE 4.3 — Some of the Alterations in Vascular Endothelium Associated With Diabetes and Hypertension

- Increased synthesis and plasma level of endothelin-1 (a vasoconstrictive substance)
- Decreased prostacyclin release (a vasodilator substance)
- Increased destruction of endothelium-derived relaxing factor (nitric oxide [NO]) and decreased responsiveness to NO
- Impaired fibrinolytic activity
- Increased endothelial cell procoagulant activity
- Increased levels of advanced glycosylated end products
- Increased superoxide anion generation

capillary endothelium; weakening of intracellular junctions; and altered protein and glycoprotein synthesis. Hyperglycemia also enhances production of the endothelial cell matrix, which may contribute to basement membrane thickening. All of these processes are of importance in the progression of atherogenesis. The enzymes involved in collagen synthesis increase when hyperglycemia is present and there is a tendency for increased thrombus formation. The increased glycation and oxidation (glycooxidation) that occur with hyperglycemia play a role in delaying endothelial cell replication and increasing cell death.

Coagulation Abnormalities in Diabetes and Hypertension

Persons with diabetes and hypertension are prone to thrombosis because of a complex interplay among enhanced coagulation factors and diminished fibrinolytic activities, enhanced platelet aggregation, and endothelial dysfunction. A procoagulant state in diabetes is mediated, in part, by higher than normal levels of several coagulation factors (**Table 4.4**).

Plasma levels of lipoprotein (a) (Lp[a]) have been reported to be elevated in diabetic patients, particularly those with poor glycemic control. By inhibiting

TABLE 4.4 — Coagulation and Fibrinolytic Abnormalities in Diabetes and Hypertension

- Elevated levels of factors VII and VIII
- Increased fibrinogen and plasminogen activator inhibitor-1 levels
- Elevated lipoprotein (a) levels
- Elevated thrombin-antithrombin complexes
- Decreased antithrombin III, protein C and S levels
- Decreased plasminogen activators and fibrinolytic activity

fibrinolysis, Lp(a) may delay thrombolysis and thus contribute to atherosclerotic plaque progression.

Inhibition of clot formation is modulated by specific factors that inhibit one or more of the clotting factors (antithrombin III, proteins C and S) and by the fibrinolytic system. In diabetic patients, fibrinolytic activity is decreased. Decreased levels of fibrinolytic factors have been found to be inversely related to glycemia as measured by glycosylated hemoglobin A_{1C} levels. Protein C antigenic levels are low in diabetic patients with poor glycemic control, and normalization of protein C occurs following good glycemic control. Coagulation abnormalities contribute to the marked propensity for hypercoagulability in the diabetic hypertensive patient.

Platelet Abnormalities in Diabetes

Platelet aggregation and adhesion are characteristically enhanced in diabetes (**Table 4.5**). The cause of this enhanced platelet reactivity is complex and incompletely understood. Whether the cause relates to increases in intracellular calcium, release of certain growth factors, serotonin, or increased destruction of

---

TABLE 4.5 — Platelet Function Abnormalities in Diabetes and Hypertension

- Increase occurs in:
  - Platelet adhesiveness and aggregation
  - Platelet generation of vasoconstrictor prostanoids
- Decrease occurs in:
  - Platelet survival
  - Platelet generation of prostacyclin and other vasodilator prostanoids
  - Platelet production of nitric oxide
- Alteration occurs in platelet divalent cation homeostasis (decreased Mg^{2+} and increased Ca^{2+})

NO, the end result is a tendency for diabetic patients to experience more clotting disorders than non-diabetics.

Microalbuminuria and CVD in Diabetes and Hypertension

There is considerable evidence that the presence of hypertension in type 1 diabetes is a consequence rather than a cause of renal disease. For example, with low levels of microalbuminuria, the BP remains normal, a finding that suggests the nephropathy precedes the rise in BP. Regardless of whether hypertension in type 1 diabetes is the etiologic factor of nephropathy or a complication of the disease, it is clear that a genetic disposition to hypertension is important in the development of nephropathy in approximately 30% of type 1 diabetics who develop this complication. It is also clear that nephropathy and hypertension accelerate each other in a logarithmic fashion.

The normal rate of protein excretion in healthy adults is <150 mg/day. Less than 30 mg of this is albumin, which has a molecular weight just large enough to keep it from passing through the normal, intact glomerulas. The remaining urine protein is comprised of different proteins and glucoproteins from tubular epithelial cells. Albumin, however, accounts for most of the protein in the urine in proteinuria due to glomerular injury, the major pathologic form of proteinuria in diabetic patients. The glomerular disease seen with diabetes is most commonly diffuse glomerulosclerosis.

The glomerular damage associated with diabetes occurs as a result of several mechanisms. One mechanism is that of glomerular capillary hypertension that leads to increased filtration and an interstitial inflammatory reaction. Glomerular capillary hypertension also increases mechanical stretch and pressure in residual glomeruli, which results in localized production of additional angiotensin II, stimulation of cytokines such as tumor growth factor-beta (TGF-β), interleukins, and plasminogen activator inhibitor-7, and a subsequent increase in collagen synthesis and scarring.

Inconsistent with the notion that glomerulosclerosis and atherosclerosis are parallel processes, early proteinuria (microalbuminuria) is associated with endothelial cell dysfunction, enhanced oxidative stress, increased inflammation, impaired fibrinolysis, elevated systolic blood pressure (SBP), nondipping, and a diabetic dyslipidemia.

Microalbuminuria, defined as 30 to 300 mg/day urinary protein, is an independent risk factor for development of CVD and a predictor of CV mortality in the diabetic population (**Figure 4.5**). It has been cor-

FIGURE 4.5 — Microalbuminuria and Ischemic Heart Disease Risk

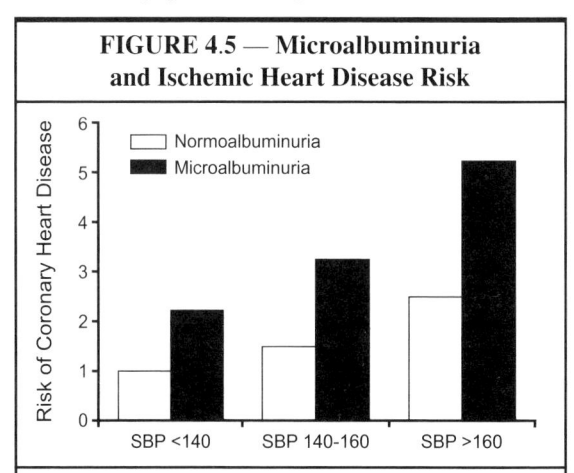

The presence of microalbuminuria (24-hour excretion of between 30 and 300 mg/d urinary protein) is associated with an increased risk of coronary heart disease at all levels of systolic blood pressure (SBP). (n = 2085; 10-year follow-up)

Borch-Johnsen K, et al. *Arterioscler Thromb Vasc Biol.* 1999;19:1992.

related with insulin resistance, atherogenic dyslipidemia, central obesity, and the absence of a nocturnal drop in both SBP and diastolic blood pressure (DBP), and it is a part of the metabolic CV syndrome associated with hypertension (Syndrome X) (**Table 4.6**). There is a strong association between microalbuminuria and insulin resistance. Microalbuminuria may precede and even predict the onset of type 2 diabetes. It is related to endothelial dysfunction and increased oxidative stress. Therefore, it is not surprising that diabetic glomerulosis parallels diabetic vascular atherosclerosis and that microalbuminuria is a powerful predictor of CHD and stroke in diabetic persons.

TABLE 4.6 — Cardiovascular Risk Factors That Tend to Cluster With Microalbuminuria

- Systolic hypertension >135 mm Hg
- Insulin resistance
- Low high-density lipoprotein cholesterol levels
- High triglyceride levels
- Central obesity
- Absent nocturnal drop in blood pressure
- Salt sensitivity
- Male gender
- Increased cardiovascular oxidative stress
- Impaired endothelial function
- Abnormal coagulation/fibrinolytic profiles

Numerous studies have linked microalbuminuria to other CVD risk factors, such as an increase in oxygen free radicals and low HDL cholesterol levels. These observations collectively indicate that microalbuminuria clusters with most of the other CVD risk factors and that it reflects generalized CV/renal endothelial dysfunction and enhanced oxidative stress.

Proteinuria appears to be a relatively strong surrogate marker for endothelial dysfunction and accelerated atherosclerosis. Patients with proteinuria have greater left ventricular mass, greater carotid medial thickening, and endothelial dysfunction. They have a greater propensity to myocardial infarction, stroke, and greater mortality with these events.

In summary, CVD is a major cause of mortality in individuals with diabetes. Many factors, including hypertension, contribute to the high prevalence of CVD in this population. Hypertension occurs approximately twice as frequently in patients with diabetes compared with patients without diabetes. Conversely, recent data suggest that hypertensive persons are more likely to develop diabetes than normotensive persons. In addition, up to 75% of CVD in patients with diabetes may be attributed to hypertension, leading to recommendations for more aggressive BP control (ie, <130/80-85 mm Hg) in persons with coexistent diabetes and hypertension. Increasing obesity further contributes to both diabetes and hypertension and significantly increases CVD morbidity and mortality.

Other important risk factors for CVD in these patients include atherosclerosis, dyslipidemia, microalbuminuria, endothelial dysfunction, platelet hyperaggregability, coagulation abnormalities, and diabetic cardiomyopathy. Both hygienic measures (weight loss and aerobic exercise) as well as treatment strategies that include aspirin, statins, insulin sensitizers, and antihypertensive agents that reduce RAAS activity have been shown to reduce inflammation, coagulation abnormalities, endothelial function, proteinuria, and in some cases, CVD and renal disease progression. Additional therapeutic agents are currently being developed to specifically improve insulin sensitivity and other CVD risk factors that are components of the cardiometabolic syndrome.

Pathologic Correlation of Proteinuria and Atherosclerosis

There are many similarities between structure and function of the vasculature and renal glomeruli. The pathophysiologic changes that occur in glomerulosclerosis are similar to those of atherosclerosis and probably are due to many of the same pathologic mechanisms. These changes include mesangial proliferation, foam-cell accumulation, appearance of extracellular matrix, deposition of amorphous debris, and eventually atherosclerosis. Oxidized LDL plays an important role in the kidney damage in patients with diabetes and hypertension. Oxidized LDL binds to substances in the glomerular membrane, which leads to increased permeability of the membrane to macrophages. Moreover, intramesangial oxidized LDL attracts the accumulation of macrophages. Thus albuminuria, which is a hallmark of glomerulosclerosis, parallels atherosclerotic changes and is predictive of increased CV mortality in diabetic patients.

As noted, microalbuminuria represents a significant risk factor for CVD both in those with clinical diabetes and in those who do not have this disorder. In population-based studies, an increased urinary albumin excretion rate (AER) has been shown to cluster with CVD risk factors. Indeed, microalbuminuria is directly related to insulin levels following an oral glucose load, and to salt sensitivity, resistance to insulin-stimulated glucose uptake, and, to reemphasize, central obesity, dyslipidemia, LVH, and the absence of nocturnal drops in both SBP and DBP. Several recent prospective studies examining progression of albuminuria in type 2 diabetes have found that elevated SBP is a significant determining factor in this progression. This is important since insulin-resistant prediabetic persons (patients with essential hypertension) as well as those with diabetes have a particular predilection toward elevated SBP. This may be related to early loss of elasticity of large vessels.

Relationships Between Microproteinuria, Glucose Metabolism, and Diabetes

Glucose metabolism, as measured by the insulin-clamp technique, has been observed to be impaired in normotensive type 2 diabetic persons with microalbuminuria compared with normotensive normoalbuminuric persons; the defect in insulin sensitivity was shown to correlate with urinary albumin excretion. The insulin clamp technique measures the amount of insulin required to maintain a near optimal level of serum glucose. Insulin resistance is measured by the amount of insulin required. Several laboratories also have found that insulin sensitivity was not diminished in healthy type 2 diabetic subjects unless microalbuminuria or hypertension or both were also present. These investigations thus add to data that establish an important link between insulin resistance and the development of microalbuminuria in persons with type 2 diabetes.

The link between insulin resistance and microalbuminuria extends to persons without clinical evidence of diabetes. A recent publication described a group of nondiabetic, normotensive, first-degree relatives of patients with type 2 diabetes mellitus who were insulin resistant and also had microalbuminuria. Persons with microalbuminuria who had not developed clinical diabetes after 3.5 years still manifested multiple CVD risk factors, including hypertension, dyslipidemia (characterized by low HDL and elevated triglycerides), and high plasma levels of insulin, all components of the insulin-resistant syndrome associated with hypertension.

Thus diabetes and hypertension are closely related to several important metabolic disorders in addition to renal factors that may be noted clinically even before a diagnosis of diabetes is made. This should heighten the awareness of physicians to intervene as early as possible in as many areas as possible when patients present with elements of the diabetes-hypertension-metabolic syndrome—lower BP, attempt to correct lipid abnormalities, employ methods to prevent clotting, and promote weight loss and exercise to decrease insulin resistance and possibly improve endothelial cell dysfunction.

The Kidney: Microalbuminuria and Progression of Renal Disease

Epidemiologic studies indicate that elevated BP, especially SBP, is associated with progression of diabetic nephropathy to end-stage renal disease (ESRD). To date, it appears that the two most important factors in preventing ESRD in diabetic patients are:
- Glucose and BP control prior to the development of diabetic nephropathy
- Rigorous BP control if evidence of nephropathy is present.

Once evidence of kidney involvement is present (>30 mg/day proteinuria), reduction of BP, especially SBP, is by far the most important intervention that can be undertaken to prevent progression of diabetic renal disease. A recent review of clinical studies on renal disease progression in diabetic patients indicated that BP reductions to levels of <130/80-85 mm Hg appear to provide protection against progression of diabetic nephropathy. There is evidence that it is important to include an ACE inhibitor or an ARB as a component of antihypertensive therapy to maximize renal protection. In most cases, the addition of a diuretic or other medication will be necessary to lower BP to goal levels.

The hallmark of diabetic glomerular disease is albuminuria. AER is normally <30 mg/day; levels >300 mg/day (200 µg/min) indicate proteinuria. Microalbuminuria is defined as persistent values of urinary albumin between 30 and 300 mg/day (20-200 µg/min). This level is not usually detectable on a dipstick test. A spot morning urine measurement of albumin and creatinine is probably the most effective ascertainment of microproteinuria. A value >0.03 indicates that albuminuria is present. The amount of creatinine is determined to indicate the percentage of the 24-hour urine excreted in the overnight specimen. Normally, the total 24-hour creatinine output is about 1.2 to 1.4 g. In diabetic patients treated with antihypertensive agents, spot morning urine albumin/creatinine should be checked at 6 months after initiating or intensifying therapy, and then generally at yearly intervals.

As a progressive increase in albuminuria is a risk factor for CVD as well as progressive nephropathy, it is a signal for more intensive antihypertensive therapy, as well as for more aggressive approaches to other risk factors (ie, lipids). Treatment strategies that have been shown to affect the progression of microalbuminuria and renal disease include both blood glucose and BP control. Recently, data that were reported from a multicenter Veterans Administration trial indicated that intensive glycemic control over a 2-year period reduced the progression to greater proteinuria but did not lessen the deterioration in creatinine clearance.

A number of clinical trials in diabetic patients have demonstrated that antihypertensive agents, particularly ACE inhibitors and ARBs (but other antihypertensive agents as well), will reduce proteinuria. A relatively recent meta-analysis of clinical trials of ACE inhibitors in diabetic patients with microalbuminuria found that, overall, ACE inhibitors reduced progression from microalbuminuria to macroalbuminuria by 79%. Further, regression to albumin-free urine occurred more than twice as often with an ACE inhibitor–based treatment strategy than with a regimen that did not include an ACE inhibitor. The effect of ACE inhibitor therapy was greatest in those with the highest AER, ranging from a 26% reduction at 20 mg/min to an 81% reduction at an AER of 200 mg/min. The treatment effect was unaltered by glycemic control, BP, gender, or age and seemed to be greater in patients with diabetes of longer duration. Three recent trials have clearly established that treatment regimens that include an ARB will decrease renal disease progression when compared with a program that does not include an ARB or ACE inhibitor (see Chapter 6 for details of these studies—Reduction of End points in Noninsulin Dependent Diabetes Mellitus With an Angiotensin II Antagonist, Losartan (RENAAL), Irbesartan Diabetic Nephropathy Trial (IDNT), and Irbesartan Microalbuminuria Type 2 Diabetes Mellitus in Hypertension Patients trial (IRMA 2).

In trials in both type 1 and type 2 diabetics, inhibition of the activity of the RAAS prevented progression of microalbuminuria and resulted in preservation of renal function. These data suggest that the diabetic patient with microalbuminuria should be treated with an ACE inhibitor or an ARB regardless of BP and that treatment should aim for normalization of albumin excretion. It should be emphasized that in all of these trials, other medications (most often a diuretic) were required to decrease BP toward a goal level. Thus the treated hypertensive patient in whom microalbuminuria persists should have their BP treatment intensified. This most often requires the use of other antihypertensive agents, particularly a diuretic. Further, given the high CVD risk in diabetic patients with microalbuminuria, concomitant therapies with lipid-lowering agents and aspirin should be initiated or intensified (**Figure 4.6**). **Table 4.7** summarizes the significance of microproteinuria and how it is measured.

FIGURE 4.6 — Association of Microalbuminuria and Cardiovascular Morbidity and Mortality in Type 2 Diabetes

Niskanen, et al (1993)
Neil, et al (1993)
Stehouwer, et al (1990)
Stiegler, et al (1992)
Patrick, et al (1990)

Subtotal

Macleod, et al (1995)

Total

0.5 1 2 5 10 20 50 100
Odds ratios of CV morbidity and mortality in patients with type 2 diabetes with microalbuminuria vs normoalbuminuria

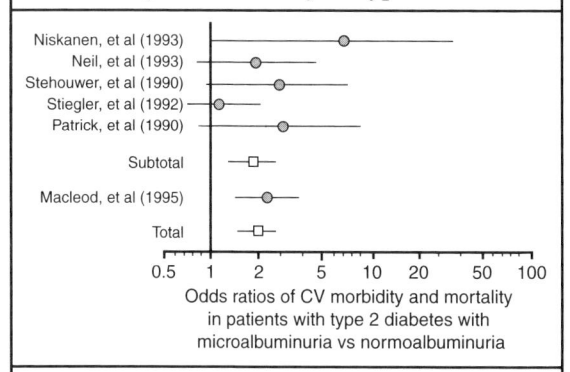

Microalbuminuria is a strong predictor of all-cause mortality and cardiovascular (CV) morbidity and mortality in type 2 diabetes. A meta-analysis of prospective trials of patients with type 2 diabetes found an overall odds ratio of 3.1 for total mortality and 1.8 for CV morbidity and mortality in patients with microproteinuria. Although the mechanism underlying the association between microalbuminuria and mortality is not clear, the presence of microalbuminuria may reflect a generalized defect in vascular permeability leading to atherogenesis. Hypertension is a major risk factor for the development of microalbuminuria.

Dinneen SF, Gerstein HC. *Arch Intern Med*. 1997;157:1413-1418.

TABLE 4.7 — Microalbuminuria

What is it?
Excretion of small amounts (30-300 mg/d) of protein in the urine

How it is determined?
Spot morning urine sample for protein (creatinine levels in the urine to determine the percentage of 24-hr urine volume excreted). Use albumin-to-creatinine ratio; >0.03 indicates proteinuria

What testing methods are available?
Micral II dipstick ($4 to $7/strip) and spot urine for albumin-to-creatinine ratio ($12 to $14/sample)

What does it mean?
Is suggestive of vascular injury not just in the kidney but in blood vessels elsewhere (correlates with cardiovascular risk)

What should be done about it?
Glycemic control; control of blood pressure (BP) to levels <130-135/80-85 mm Hg

Is specific therapy indicated?
The use of an angiotensin-converting enzyme inhibitor or an angiotensin II receptor blocker usually with a diuretic; probably represents the most appropriate therapy to lower BP and reduce proteinuria

SELECTED READING

Bakins G. Microproteinuria. What is it? Why is it important? What should be done about it? *J Clin Hypertens*. 2001;3:99-103.

Capes SE, Gerstein HC, Negassa A, Yusuf S. Enalapril prevents clinical proteinuria in diabetic patients with low ejection fraction. *Diabetes Care*. 2000;23:377-380.

Chaturvedi N, Sjolie AK, Stephenson JM, et al. Effect of lisinopril on progression of retinopathy in normotensive people with type 1 diabetes. The EUCLID Study Group. EURODIAB controlled trial of lisinopril in insulin-dependent diabetes mellitus. *Lancet*. 1998;351:28-31.

Dinneen SF, Gerstein HC. The association of microalbuminuria and mortality in non–insulin-dependent diabetes mellitus. A systemic overview of the literature. *Arch Intern Med*. 1997;157:1413-1418.

Forsblom CM, Eriksson JG, Ekstrand AV, Teppo AM, Taskinen MR, Groop LC. Insulin resistance and abnormal albumin excretion in non-diabetic first-degree relatives of patients with NIDDM. *Diabetologia*. 1995;38:363-369.

Hypertension in Diabetes Study Group. Hypertension in Diabetes Study (HDS):1. Prevalence of hypertension in newly presenting type 2 diabetic patients and the association with risk factors for cardiovascular and diabetic complications. *J Hypertens*. 1993;11:309-317.

Kuusisto J, Mykkanen L, Pyorala K, Laakson M. Hyperinsulinemic microalbuminuria. A new risk indicator for coronary heart disease. *Circulation*. 1995;91:831-837.

Lewis EJ, Hunsicker LG, Bain RP, Rohde RD. The effect of angiotensin-converting-enzyme inhibition on diabetic nephropathy. The Collaborative Study Group. *N Engl J Med*. 1993;329:1456-1462.

O'Driscoll G, Green D, Rankin J, Stanton K, Taylor R. Improvement in endothelial function by angiotensin converting enzyme inhibition in insulin-dependent diabetes mellitus. *J Clin Invest*. 1997;100:678-684.

Sowers JR. Insulin and insulin-like growth factor in normal and pathological cardiovascular physiology. *Hypertension*. 1997;29:691-699.

Sowers JR. Insulin resistance and hypertension. *Am J Physiol Heart Circ Physiol*. 2004;286:H1597-H1602.

Velloso LA, Folli F, Sun XJ, White MF, Saad MJ, Kahn CR. Cross-talk between insulin and angiotensin signaling systems. *Proc Natl Acad Sci USA*. 1996;93:12490-12495.

5 The Renin-Angiotensin-Aldosterone System in Diabetes

Hypertension is a major component of the metabolic cardiovascular (CV)/metabolic syndrome in diabetes. Insulin resistance plays an important role in promoting hypertension in patients with this syndrome. The renin-angiotensin-aldosterone system (RAAS) also appears to play an important role in the development of hypertension in diabetic patients. It exerts its hypertensive action via stimulation of salt and water retention, increasing vascular tone and interference with the vasorelaxing action of insulin. Effects of the RAAS are not limited to regulation of vascular tone but are much more pleiotropic. This system is necessary to sustain CV function, particularly with relation to maintaining plasma volume. Chronic overactivity, however, leads to maladaptive tissue responses such as a permanent increase of vascular resistance, myocardial fibrosis and hypertrophy, endothelial dysfunction, decreased stability of atherosclerotic plaques, and reduced fibrinolysis/increased coagulation.

The angiotensin-converting enzyme (ACE) is a key enzyme in the activation of the RAAS, which helps to convert angiotensin I (an inactive substance) to angiotensin II. In addition, it inactivates vasodilatory kinins (such as bradykinin) (**Figure 5**.**1**). Angiotensin II and aldosterone are major hormones that exert their actions to maintain fluid volume and promote increased vasomotor tone. They are produced by the heart, kidney, and the vasculature where they have local actions. ACE inhibitors block the generation of angiotensin II and increase the availability of vasodilat-

FIGURE 5.1—Site of Action of ACE Inhibitors and Angiotensin II Receptor Blockers

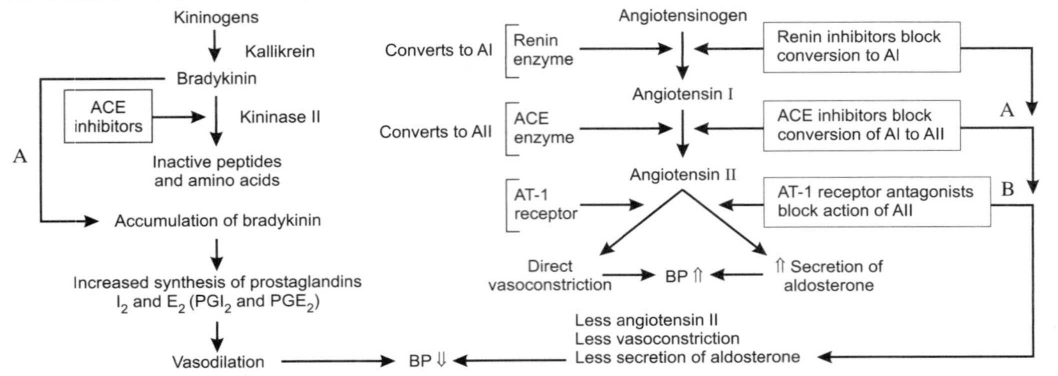

(A) Mode of action of angiotensin-converting enzyme (ACE) inhibitors: block conversion of angiotensin I (AI) (an inactive substance) to AII (a vasoconstrictor). This action (1) decreases the generation of AII, and also by blocking the activity of kininase II, (2) decreases the breakdown of bradykinin; this vasodilator substance increases and blood pressure (BP) is lowered. (B) Mode of action of angiotensin II receptor blocker (AT-1): blocks effects of AII peripherally; aldosterone secretion is not increased and vasoconstriction is prevented; *no effect on bradykinin system*. Does not prevent production of angiotensin II.

ing substances such as bradykinin. There are several angiotensin II receptors: AT_1 is the major receptor controlling vasomotor tone and is the receptor inhibited by the angiotensin II receptor blockers (ARBs). The relationship between RAAS and insulin signaling is complex and involves several intracellular mechanisms and signaling pathways.

Normally, insulin binds to its receptor on the surface of insulin-sensitive cells and triggers a series of reactions in insulin receptor substances that aid in glucose transport. Activation of the angiotensin II (AT_1 receptor) decreases insulin's ability to stimulate glucose transport; this leads to insulin resistance (more insulin is required to maintain a stable serum glucose level). ACE inhibitor therapy improves insulin sensitivity, in part, by overcoming some of these effects of angiotensin II on insulin-stimulated glucose transport in skeletal muscle tissue. ARBs are also effective in reducing the activity of angiotensin II in peripheral tissues.

Cardiomyopathy, one of the complications of diabetes, is probably linked to activation of local RAAS in the heart. Angiotensinogen, renin, and AT_1 receptor concentrations are increased in the heart of diabetic animals. This increased RAAS expression in the heart leads to increased fibrosis, altered nitric oxide (NO) metabolism, reduced sodium pump and potassium channel expression/activity, and delayed diastolic relaxation that characterizes diabetic cardiomyopathy. These observations may also explain why ACE inhibitor and aldosterone antagonism have been so beneficial in diabetic patients with cardiovascular disease (CVD). ACE inhibitors appear to exert beneficial effects on both left ventricular diastolic and systolic function in diabetics. Improved cardiac function also influences the rate of albumin excretion in patients with overt or preclinical diabetic nephropathy.

ACE inhibitors also protect against deterioration of renal function in diabetic nephropathy and their use may produce benefits over and above blood pressure (BP) control alone. In the Heart Outcomes Prevention Evaluation and Microalbuminuria, Cardiovascular, and Renal Outcomes (MICRO-HOPE) study, a dose of ramipril (an ACE inhibitor) 10 mg/day in addition to other medications lowered the risk of overt nephropathy by 24% in a group of very high-risk patients compared with subjects who did not receive ACE inhibitor therapy. These results indicate that ACE inhibitor therapy may be particularly beneficial in diabetic patients who have cardiac and renal disease. Recent data suggest that ARBs have a similar action. As noted, the use of a β-blocker/diuretic treatment program will also reduce proteinuria and at least in one trial (United Kingdom Prospective Diabetes Study [UKPDS]), these therapies were as effective in reducing morbidity/mortality as an ACE inhibitor program in diabetic patients (if BP control was achieved) (see Chapter 6, *Results of Hypertension Treatment Trials in Diabetic Patients*).

Effect of ACE Inhibition on Insulin Resistance and the Development of New-Onset Diabetes

The Captopril Prevention Project (CAPPP) was the first interventional randomized study that showed that ACE inhibitors might actually prevent the development of clinical diabetes. It further showed that the group of hypertensive patients treated with captopril, an ACE inhibitor, had a significantly lower rate of development of new-onset diabetes (NOD) compared with the group of patients receiving conventional therapy.

During the 5-year follow-up period of the Heart Outcomes Prevention Evaluation (HOPE) trial, there was a 34% reduction in the development of NOD in patients receiving the ACE inhibitor compared with the non–ACE inhibitor-treated group. *In all of the trials in hypertensive diabetes, multiple medications were usually necessary to lower BP to goal levels.* In most of the trials, a large percentage of patients were receiving a diuretic in addition to the study drugs.

Studies have shown that ACE inhibitors increase insulin sensitivity and improve glycemic control in patients with clinical diabetes mellitus. The results of the MICRO-HOPE trial showed that diabetic patients taking ramipril (plus other medications) had better-controlled diabetes than patients taking medications that did not include an ACE inhibitor. Compared with baseline, mean absolute glycosylated hemoglobin (HbA_{1C}) values were 1.5% higher than the upper limit of normal in the ramipril group and 3.4% in the other group at 1 year. At 2 years, HbA_{1C} decreased by 0.1% in participants taking ramipril and rose by 2.2% in participants taking other medications that did not include an ACE inhibitor. Similar results were reported by the EURODIAB Controlled Trial of Lisinopril in Insulin-Dependent Diabetes Mellitus (EUCLID) study, which showed that HbA_{1C} was significantly lower in a lisinopril (ACE inhibitor)–treated group than in a placebo group. An increased incidence of hypoglycemia has been reported in diabetic patients receiving a combination of an ACE inhibitor and oral hypoglycemic agents or insulin. These clinical results suggest that ACE inhibitor therapy increases insulin sensitivity in people with insulin resistance: this would include patients with essential hypertension.

The mechanism by which ACE inhibitors improve insulin sensitivity in patients with diabetes, hypertension, and the metabolic CV syndrome is complex and not completely understood. It likely involves an improvement in blood flow to insulin-resistant muscles and enhancement of insulin signaling at the cellular level. Moreover, ACE inhibitors have an ability to reduce the free fatty acid (FFA) levels in insulin-resistant animal models; this would decrease the FFA-glucose cycle and therefore increase insulin sensitivity.

It has been observed that ACE inhibitors are able to facilitate blood flow through the microcirculation in skeletal muscles. This effect is bradykinin-dependent and realized through activation of cell-surface receptors. As noted in **Figure 5.1**, ACE inhibitor therapy prolongs the action of bradykinin by blocking its enzymatic breakdown and facilitating its action on receptors. Bradykinin not only causes vasodilation but also independently increases the basal and insulin-stimulated rate of glucose uptake in skeletal muscle in insulin-resistant states. Thus ACE inhibitors may mediate improvements in insulin actions, at least in part, through bradykinin-mediated mechanisms. This specific action on bradykinin is not seen following the use of an ARB, which does not interfere with its degradation.

A review of data on the occurrence of NOD in hypertensive patients treated with antihypertensive medications indicates the following:

- Hypertensives develop diabetes more frequently than normotensive individuals.
- The use of diuretics compared with placebo may increase NOD by approximately 1% (about 1.2/1000 patient years) (**Table 5.1**).
- β-Blockers increase NOD by about 7.3/1000 patient years compared with no therapy.
- Comparative clinical trials with different medications where patient populations vary considerably indicate that agents that block the RAAS system (eg, ACE inhibitors and ARBs) decrease the occurrence of NOD by about 2% to 3% compared with treatments that did not include these agents (**Table 5.2** and **Table 5.3**).

These data add to the recommendation that in obese subjects or patients with manifestations of the metabolic syndrome, a RAAS inhibitor should be part of the treatment program.

ACE Inhibitors and Vascular Health in the Diabetic Patient With Hypertension

To reemphasize, ACE inhibitors reduce oxidation of low-density lipoprotein (LDL), decrease fibrinogen levels, reduce oxidative stress, and normalize endothelial NO function both by increased production and by decreased destruction of NO. Improvement of insulin-mediated vascular relaxation is noted. Moreover, ACE inhibition decreases secretion of endothelin-1, which is a potent vasoconstrictor and a mitogenic factor for vascular smooth muscle cells and fibroblasts via bradykinin, and therefore an NO-dependent mechanism. ACE inhibitors may also diminish expression of adhesion molecules by the endothelium and decrease cytokine-induced inflammation, both of which are important in the atherogenic process that is enhanced in diabetic vasculature.

Several trials have indicated that in patients with diabetes and hypertension, ACE inhibitors appear to be superior to other treatment modalities in terms of reduction of risk of CVD events and may provide benefit above that offered by reduction of BP alone. In the HOPE study in very high-risk patients who were on multiple medications, the addition of an ACE inhibitor (ramipril) lowered the risk of myocardial infarction (MI) by 22%, stroke by 33%, CV mortality by 24%, and total mortality by 24%. All of these changes were achieved by a mechanism probably other than BP lowering since BP differences between the ACE-inhibitor–treated group and a control group were

TABLE 5.1 — Effects of Moderate- and High-Dose Diuretic Therapy on Glucose Metabolism in Placebo-Controlled Trials

Study	Duration/Years	Serum Glucose (mg/dL)	Hyperglycemia or Diabetes
Oslo	5	No difference—diuretics; placebo	No specific data available
EWPHE	3	Increase 6.6—diuretics; placebo	Excess of 6/1000 patient years
MRC	3	No specific data available	Excess of 6/1000 patient years
HAPPHY	4	No specific data available	Excess of 6/1000 patient years
HDFP	5	No specific data available	1.6% (57/3563)
SHEP	3	Difference of 4 mg/dL—drug vs placebo in diabetics Difference of 3 mg/dL in nondiabetics	1 of 483 No significant difference in number of new cases of diabetes in treatment group compared with placebo group
MRFIT	6	No specific data available	Excess of 7%—special intervention group with diuretics vs excess of 2%—usual care group without diuretics*

ALLHAT	at 4+ years	Increase of 3 mg/dL (ACE inhibitor ↓ 1 mg/dL)	3.5% more new-onset diabetes with diuretics compared with ACE inhibitors[†]
VA	2	Increase of 1.7—diuretics; placebo	No specific data available
TOMHS	1	Decrease of 0.9—diuretics Decrease of 3.2—placebo	No specific data available

Abbreviations: ACE, angiotensin-converting enzyme; ALLHAT, Antihypertensive and Lipid-Lowering Treatment to Prevent Heart Attack Trial; EWPHE, European Working Party on High Blood Pressure in the Elderly; HAPPHY, Heart Attack Primary Prevention in Hypertension; HDFP, Hypertension Detection and Follow-up Program; MRC, Medical Research Council; MRFIT, Multiple Risk Factor Intervention Trial; SHEP, Systolic Hypertension in the Elderly Program; TOMHS, Treatment of Mild Hypertension Study; VA, Veterans Administration single-drug therapy for hypertension in men.

[*] Fasting glucose ≥110 mg/dL.
[†] Fasting glucose >126 mg/dL.

Modified and updated from: *Cleve Clin J Med.* 1993;60:27-37.

TABLE 5.2 — New-Onset Diabetes in the Prospective, Comparative, Randomized Hypertension Treatment Trials (3-to-8 Years Follow-Up)*

Trial (No. Patients)	Duration/Years	Therapy	New-Onset Diabetes (%)	Absolute Difference (%)
ALLHAT (21,294)	5+	Diuretic ACE-I CCB	11.6 ⎤ 8.1 ⎦ 9.8 ⎦	— 3.5 1.8
ANBP-2 (5626)	4+	Diuretic ACE-I	6.56 4.54	2.02
CAPPP (10,985)	6+	β-Bl and diuretic ACE-I	7.3 6.5	0.8
CHARM (5439)	3+	Other therapy (UC) ARB	7.4 6.0	1.4
HOPE (5720)	5	Other therapy (UC) ACE-I	5.4 3.6	1.8

INSIGHT (5019)	4+	Diuretic CCB	7.0 5.4	1.6
INVEST (16,176)	5+	β-Bl and diuretic CCB/ACE-I	8.2 7.0	1.2
LIFE (7998)	5	β-Bl ARB	8.0 6.0	2.0
SCOPE (4342)	5	Other therapy (UC) ARB	5.3 4.3	1.0
STOP-2 (5895)	6+	UC CCB ACE-I	4.9 4.8 4.7	— 0.01 0.02
VALUE (15,245)	4+	ARB CCB	13.1 16.4	3.3

Continued

Abbreviations: ACE-I, angiotensin-converting enzyme inhibitor; ALLHAT, Antihypertensive and Lipid-Lowering Treatment to Prevent Heart Attack Trial; ANBP, Australian National Blood Pressure; ARB, angiotensin II receptor blocker; β-Bl, β-blocker; CAPPP, Captopril Prevention Project; CCB, calcium channel blocker; CHARM, Candesartan in Heart Failure—Assessment of Reduction in Mortality and Morbidity; HOPE, Heart Outcomes Prevention Evaluation; INSIGHT, International Nifedipine Gastrointestinal Therapeutic System Study Intervention as a Goal for Hypertension Therapy; INVEST, International Verapamil SR/Trandolapril Study; LIFE, Losartan Intervention for End-point Reduction in Hypertension; SCOPE, Study on Cognition and Prognosis in the Elderly; STOP, Swedish Trial in Older Patients With Hypertension; UC, usual care; VALUE, Valsartan Antihypertensive Long-term Use Evaluation.

* Multiple medications used in all trials in an effort to achieve goal blood pressure levels; >100,000 patients.

only 2.4 mm Hg systolic and 1.0 mm Hg diastolic. Some experts believe that a difference of even this magnitude may account for at least some of the benefit of treatment. In addition, there is some question that in the HOPE trial, when the study drug was given in the evening, the nighttime BPs were considerably lower in this cohort (based on a very small subject of patients who were studied with ambulatory BP monitoring).

As reviewed in Chapter 6, a meta-analysis of several randomized controlled trials (Appropriate Blood Pressure Control in Diabetes [ABCD], Fosinopril vs Amlodipine Cardiovascular Event Trial [FACET], and CAPPP) that included a total of 2,180 patients with type 2 diabetes and hypertension treated with ACE inhibitors compared with another antihypertensive agent(s) showed a benefit of ACE inhibitors compared with alternative treatment in the outcomes of acute MI (63% reduction), CVD events (51% reduction), and all-cause mortality (62% reduction). The ABCD trial was terminated early after the superiority of ACE inhibition over calcium channel blockade was established. The FACET was originally designed to compare the effects of fosinopril vs amlodipine on serum lipid levels and diabetic control in 380 patients with type 2 diabetes and hypertension. Even though there were no differences in glucose and lipid control in the two groups by the end of 3.5 years of follow-up, subjects assigned to fosinopril treatment were at significantly lower risk for the combined outcome of stroke, MI, and hospitalization for angina than subjects assigned to amlodipine treatment. It should be noted that patients treated with both fosinopril and amlodipine had the least CVD events. The numbers of patients with defined end points were small in both the ABCD trial and FACET.

To recap another study (UKPDS) that compared outcomes of treatment with an ACE inhibitor

TABLE 5.3 — Incidence of New-Onset Diabetes With Different Antihypertensive Medications in the 3-to-8 Year Hypertension Treatment Trials

Trial	Therapy	Duration (Years)	New-Onset Diabetes (%)		Absolute Difference (%)
			ACE-I	UC or D/β-Bl	
ACE-I Compared With Usual Care (D/β-Bl)					
CAPPP	ACE-I/β-Bl/D	6.1	6.5	7.5	1.0
STOP-2	ACE-I/β-Bl/D	6+	4.7	4.9	0.2
ANBP-2	ACE-I/D	4+	4.5	6.6	2.1
ALLHAT	ACE-I/D	4.9	8.1	11.6	3.5
			CCB	CT	
CCB Compared With Usual Care					
NORDIL	CCB/β-Bl/D	4.5	4.3	4.9	0.6
ALLHAT	CCB/D	4.9	9.8	11.6	1.8
INVEST	CCB/β-Bl	4.0	6.2	7.3	1.1
INSIGHT	CCB/D	3.5	5.4	7.0	1.6
STOP-2	CCB/β-Bl/D	6+	4.8	4.9	0.1

ARB Compared With Other Therapies				
VALUE	ARB/CCB	4.2	13.1	16.4	3.3
LIFE	ARB/β-Bl	4.8	6.0	8.0	2.0
SCOPE	ARB/UC	5	4.3	5.3	1.0
CHARM	ARB/OT	3+	6.0	7.4	1.4
ACE-I Compared With CCB			ACE-I	CCB	
ALLHAT	ACE-I/CCB	4.9	8.1	9.8	1.7

Approximate overall difference: ACE or ARB vs D/β-Bl = 2.0%; ACE vs CCB = 2.0%; CCB vs D/β-Bl = 1.5%

Abbreviations: ACE-I, angiotensin-converting enzyme inhibitor; ALLHAT, Antihypertensive and Lipid-Lowering Treatment to Prevent Heart Attack Trial; ANBP, Australian National Blood Pressure; ARB, angiotensin II receptor blocker; β-Bl, β-blocker; CAPPP, Captopril Prevention Project; CCB, calcium channel blocker; CHARM, Candesartan in Heart Failure—Assessment of Reduction in Mortality and Morbidity; CT, conventional therapy; D, diuretic; INSIGHT, International Nifedipine Gastrointestinal Therapeutic System Study Intervention as a Goal for Hypertension Therapy; INVEST, International Verapamil SR/ Trandolapril Study; LIFE, Losartan Intervention for Endpoint Reduction in Hypertension; NORDIL, Nordic Diltiazem; OT, other therapy; SCOPE, Study on Cognition and Prognosis in the Elderly; STOP, Swedish Trial in Older Patients With Hypertension; UC, usual care; VALUE, Valsartan Antihypertensive Long-term Use Evaluation.

Moser M. *J Clin Hyper*. 2004;6:610–613.

(captopril)–based treatment program vs treatment with a β-blocker (atenolol)–based treatment program, both treatment regimens were found to be equally effective in reduction of CV mortality if strict BP control was maintained. The absence of a difference in the rate of reduction of CV mortality could be explained by the similarity of action of both medications in reducing activity of the RAAS, respectively (ie, β-blockers decrease renin production; ACE inhibitors decrease angiotensin II production). ACE inhibitors favorably affect microvascular complications of diabetes, such as nephropathy and retinopathy. In the UKPDS study, as noted, these complications were also benefited equally in the β-blocker and ACE groups. Moreover, improvement in retinopathy was observed even in normotensive diabetics treated with an ACE inhibitor. It is possible, but not as yet proven in long-term studies, that the use of ARBs that block the effects of angiotensin II peripherally at the vascular receptor site might result in the same beneficial effects on CV morbidity and mortality as the ACE inhibitors. Thus far, as noted, the use of ARBs has been shown to slow down progression of renal disease in long-term studies of type 2 diabetics with varying degrees of nephropathy.

Thus ACE inhibitors or agents that block the activity of the RAAS system influence different aspects of vascular health in the patient with diabetes and hypertension. They act on almost all chains of the metabolic CV syndrome such as:

- Inhibition of the RAAS, which can improve insulin sensitivity
- Normalizing BP
- Decreasing oxidation of lipoproteins
- Restoring endothelial function.

In patients with diabetes and those with impaired glucose tolerance, ACE inhibition improves glycemic control, reduces microalbuminuria, and improves renal function. In addition, ACE inhibition is able to oppose the effect of locally activated RAAS and improve diabetic cardiomyopathy. All of the above suggest that medications that interfere with the RAAS are important in the management of diabetes and the metabolic syndrome with a potential to reduce all causes of mortality in this high-risk group. Ongoing clinical trials with ARBs and aldosterone antagonists may add additional information about improving renal and CV disease outcomes in patients with the comorbid conditions of diabetes and hypertension.

SELECTED READING

Chaturvedi N, Sjolie AK, Stephenson JM, et al. Effect of lisinopril on progression of retinopathy in normotensive people with type 1 diabetes. The EUCLID Study Group. EURODIAB controlled trial of lisinopril in insulin-dependent diabetes mellitus. *Lancet*. 1998;351:28-31.

Fiordaliso F, Li B, Latini R, et al. Myocyte death in streptozotocin-induced diabetes in rats is angiotensin II-dependent. *Lab Invest*. 2000;80:513-527.

Heart Outcomes Prevention Evaluation Study Investigators. Effect of ramipril on cardiovascular and microvascular outcomes in people with diabetes mellitus: results of the HOPE study and MICRO-HOPE substudy. Heart Outcomes Prevention Evaluation Study Investigators. *Lancet*. 2000;355:253-259.

Herings RM, de Boer A, Stricker BH, Leufkens HG, Porsius A. Hypoglycaemia associated with use of inhibitors of angiotensin converting enzyme. *Lancet*. 1995;345:1195-1198.

Mathiesen ER, Hommel E, Hansen HP, Smidt UM, Parving HH. Randomised controlled trial of long term efficacy of captopril on preservation of kidney function in normotensive patients with insulin dependent diabetes and microalbuminuria. *BMJ*. 1999;319:24-25.

McFarlane SI, Banerji M, Sowers JR. Insulin resistance and cardiovascular disease. *J Clin Endocrinol Metab*. 2001;86:713-718.

Moser M. Current hypertension management: separating fact from fiction. *Cleve Clin J Med*. 1993;60:27-37.

Moser M. New-onset diabetes in the hypertension treatment trials: a point of view. *J Clin Hyper*. 2004;6:610-613.

Muirhead N, Feagan BF, Mahon J, et al. The effects of valsartan and captopril on reducing microalbuminuria in patients with type 2 diabetes mellitus: a placebo-controlled trial. *Curr Therapeutic Res*. 1999;60:650-660.

Rachmani R, Lidar M, Brosh D, Levi Z, Ravid M. Oxidation of low-density lipoprotein in normotensive type 2 diabetic patients. Comparative effect of enalapril versus nifedipine: a randomized crossover study. *Diabetes Res Clin Pract*. 2000;48:139-145

Sowers JR. Treatment of hypertension in patients with diabetes. *Arch Intern Med*. 2004;164:1850-1857.

Young M, Funder JW. Aldosterone and the heart. *Trends Endocrinol Metab*. 2000;11:224-226.

6 Results of Hypertension Treatment Trials in Diabetic Patients

In view of unequivocal epidemiologic evidence that the risk of cardiovascular disease (CVD) is greatly increased in diabetics, evidence that has been available for >20 to 30 years, it would have seemed logical that greater efforts to reduce CVD risk factors in addition to correcting abnormal glucose metabolism might have been undertaken years ago. This is especially true in relation to hypertension. But without long-term clinical evidence that treating hypertensive diabetic patients was beneficial, many physicians were reluctant to treat patients with diabetes with antihypertensive medications or to predict with any degree of accuracy how much benefit would accrue. In many of the early hypertension studies, diabetic patients were actually excluded from treatment for fear that some of the medications might adversely affect outcome.

Definitive evidence is now available that lowering blood pressure (BP) will reduce morbidity and mortality in the diabetic patient, probably to a greater extent than controlling blood glucose levels. The evidence strongly suggests that in the young or old, man or woman, treatment of elevated BP and lowering it to goals below those set in nondiabetic patients will be beneficial. Goal BP levels in a nondiabetic are presently set at <140/90 mm Hg; goal levels in a diabetic should be set at about 130/80-85 mm Hg (**Figure 7.1**).

Early Clinical Trials in Diabetic Patients With Hypertension

■ Hypertension Detection Follow-Up Program and the Systolic Hypertension in the Elderly Program

In some earlier studies, ie, the Hypertension Detection Follow-up Program (HDFP) and in the Systolic Hypertension in the Elderly Program (SHEP), diabetes was not an exclusion criterion. In the HDFP trial, approximately 10% of the hypertensive participants were diabetics. The HDFP was a population-based trial to assess the efficacy of an intensive stepped-care (SC) antihypertensive regimen compared with community referred care (RC) among persons with diastolic hypertension (>90 mm Hg) in preventing all-cause mortality. Initial therapy in the SC group was chlorthalidone 25 mg, which could be increased to 100 mg (a dose considered unnecessarily high at present but one which was in common use in the 1960s and 1970s). Add-on therapy included a β-blocker or reserpine and other medications (eg, hydralazine, a vasodilator) that might be necessary to reduce BP. In the RC group, diuretics and other agents were also used but presumably in lower doses.

The difference in BP between the SC and the RC groups at the end of a 5-year study was –12/–5 mm Hg. A large number of subjects did not achieve the goal diastolic blood pressure (DBP) of ≤90 mm Hg. Of the more than 10,000 patients aged 30 to 69 randomized at baseline, 1079 were classified as diabetics. These included both insulin- and non–insulin-treated patients (type 1 and type 2). The diagnosis was based on a history of a fasting blood glucose of >140 mg/dL (7.8 mmol/L). This diagnostic criterion has recently been changed to fasting glucose levels of >126 mg/dL. Obviously, more patients would have been included if this newer definition had been used. At the end of 5 years in the nondiabetic group, the all-cause mortality rate was 17% lower in the SC group compared with the RC group. Overall, in diabetic patients, the death rate was similar for the SC and the RC groups (**Table 6.1**), but there were differences in outcome depending on the severity of the hypertension. A large HDFP subgroup had less severe degrees of hypertension (stage 1), defined at that time as a DBP 90-104 mm Hg (when the HDFP began, physicians paid less attention to systolic blood pressure [SBP]). More recently, stage 1 DBP has been defined as 90-100 mm Hg. In this group of less-severe hypertensives, 466 were diabetic. All-cause mortality was lower in the SC group of less-severe hypertensives than in the RC group for both diabetic and nondiabetic patients (20.5% and 22%, respectively) (**Table 6.1**).

TABLE 6.1 — Hypertension Detection and Follow-Up Program Results in Diabetic Subjects*

	Nondiabetics	Diabetics
5-y all-cause mortality	17% lower in SC group	No difference between SC and RC groups
Patients with DBPs 90-104 mm Hg (466 patients)	22.2% lower in SC group	20.5% lower in SC group[†]

Abbreviations: DBP, diastolic blood pressure; RC, referred care; SC, stepped care.

* 1079 patients with history of diabetes or fasting blood sugar ≥140 mg/dL
† Although the relative decrease in mortality was similar in the diabetic subjects, the baseline absolute risk was greater in diabetic subjects and absolute benefits were greater in those individuals.

It is well known that the outlook for untreated hypertensive diabetic patients is considerably less favorable than for nondiabetic hypertensive individuals. *At similar levels of BP; there is an increased morbidity/ mortality in untreated hypertensive diabetics compared with nondiabetics with similar elevations of BP.* Thus while the relative risk of mortality was reduced equally by about 20% to 22% in diabetics and nondiabetics who received more aggressive therapy compared with less aggressive treatment, the absolute risk reduction was greater in the diabetic patients because of the greater baseline risk.

These findings of benefit in this subgroup of SC diabetic patients with initial DBP of 90-104 mm Hg are similar to the SHEP findings. SHEP was a study of more than 5000 people >60 years of age with isolated systolic hypertension (ISH), defined at that time as SBP >160 mm Hg and a DBP ≤90 mm Hg. There were 583 patients (12%) with diabetes. This included patients with a history of diabetes, patients on oral hypoglycemic agents, and patients with fasting serum glucose levels >140 mg/dL. In this study, chlorthalidone (12.5 to 25 mg/day) was the initial drug of choice with atenolol (25 to 50 mg/day) added if necessary. The treated group consisted of 283 patients; 300 patients were given a placebo.

At the end of year 4, only about one third of the treated patients were receiving both chlorthalidone and another agent, usually atenolol. In the diabetic patients, BP was lowered by –10/2 mm Hg in the treated compared with the placebo group. At the end of the treatment period in diabetic patients, there was a significant reduction of 56% in all major coronary heart disease (CHD) events. This compares with a reduction of 19% in the treated nondiabetic patients compared with those who received placebo (**Figure 6.1**). Nonfatal myocardial infarction (MI) and fatal CHD events were also reduced significantly more in the treated dia-

> **FIGURE 6.1 — Systolic Hypertension in the Elderly Program: Influence of Diabetes on Cardiovascular Event Rates** 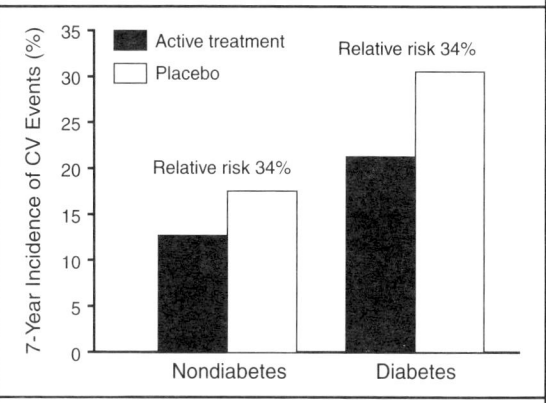
>
> [Bar chart showing 7-Year Incidence of CV Events (%) for Nondiabetes and Diabetes groups, comparing Active treatment vs Placebo. Relative risk 34% shown for both groups.]
>
> Among the 583 patients with type 2 diabetes, the 5-year major cardiovascular (CV) event rate was lower by 34% with antihypertensive therapy compared with placebo. Although an identical 34% reduction in the major CV event rate was found in nondiabetic patients, the absolute risk reduction with active treatment vs placebo was twice as great in patients with diabetes as in those without diabetes, due to the higher absolute risk of a CV event in patients with diabetes.
>
> Curb JD, et al. *JAMA*. 1996;276:1886-1892.

betic patients than in nondiabetics compared with the placebo groups; a reduction in risk of 54% in the diabetic patients and 23% in the nondiabetics compared with subjects receiving placebo. All-cause mortality was also reduced to a greater degree (26%) in the treated diabetic patients (compared with placebo) compared with 15% in the nondiabetic treated patients (compared with placebo). Fatal and nonfatal strokes, however, appeared to be reduced more in the nondiabetic cohort (**Table 6.2**): a nonsignificant reduction of –22% from placebo in diabetics and a significant re-

TABLE 6.2 — Cumulative 5-Year Rates (1000 Patient Years) of Cardiovascular Events in the Systolic Hypertension in the Elderly Program

Cardiovascular Event	Diabetic Group		Nondiabetic Group	
	Active Therapy	*Placebo*	*Active Therapy*	*Placebo*
Major coronary heart disease events	9.2	16	6.9	7.6
Nonfatal myocardial infarction or fatal coronary heart disease	7.7	13.1	5.1	5.7
Nonfatal and fatal strokes	9.7	14.4	4.4	7.5
Major cerebrovascular disease events	21.4	31.5	13.3	10.4

Placebo-treated diabetic patients had about 2 to 3 times the risk of a cardiovascular event as placebo-treated nondiabetics.

duction of –38% in nondiabetics compared with placebo. Reduction in all major CVD events was equal for treated diabetics and nondiabetic subjects (–34%) (**Figure 6.2**).

For all outcomes, the relative risk or reduction in events for treated diabetics patients was as favorable or more favorable than for treated nondiabetic patients. As noted earlier, since risk from hypertension is considerably higher in diabetic subjects, the absolute risk reductions with active treatment compared with placebo were consistently greater in treated diabetic patients than in treated nondiabetic patients; 101/1000 compared with 51/1000 randomized participants, re-

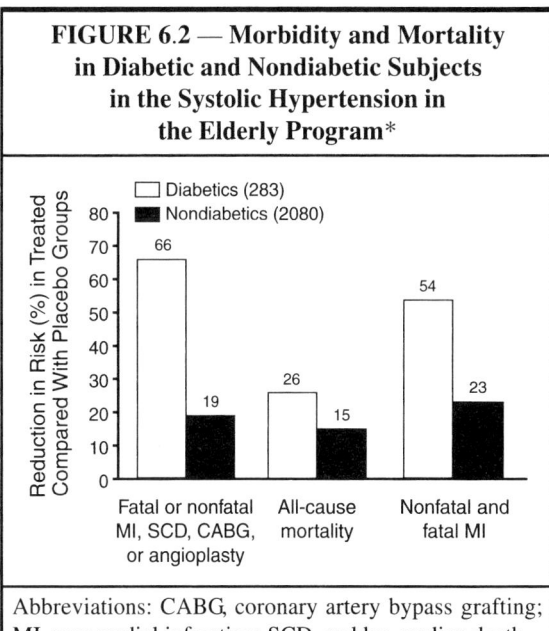

FIGURE 6.2 — Morbidity and Mortality in Diabetic and Nondiabetic Subjects in the Systolic Hypertension in the Elderly Program*

Reduction in Risk (%) in Treated Compared With Placebo Groups

- Diabetics (283)
- Nondiabetics (2080)

Outcome	Diabetics	Nondiabetics
Fatal or nonfatal MI, SCD, CABG, or angioplasty	66	19
All-cause mortality	26	15
Nonfatal and fatal MI	54	23

Abbreviations: CABG, coronary artery bypass grafting; MI, myocardial infarction; SCD, sudden cardiac death.

* Therapy: low-dose diuretic with β-blocker added if necessary; n = 4736; subjects >60 years of age.

Curb JD, et al. *JAMA*. 1996;276:1886-1892.

spectively, benefited from treatment at the 5-year follow-up. This reflects the higher baseline risk for diabetic hypertensive patients. For example, untreated diabetics had a cumulative 5-year rate of major coronary heart disease events of 16/100; untreated nondiabetics, a rate of only 7.6/100. Rates for nonfatal MI or fatal CHD were 13.1/100 compared with 5.7/100. *Therapy reduced the risk in diabetics in many categories to levels close to those in nondiabetic subjects.* In the nondiabetic group, lowering BP also reduced risk compared with risk in subjects with higher BP.

There was little or no evidence that adverse effects of treatment had impacted the important positive results in this randomized trial. Several adverse effects of therapy appeared to be more common in diabetics than in nondiabetics (**Table 6.3**). For example, cold or numb hands occurred in 25% of treated diabetics compared with 17% in the placebo group. Treated nondiabetics noted this symptom in 17% compared with 14% in the placebo group. It is recognized that sexual dysfunction, which is presumably secondary to vascular disease as well as autonomic nerve dysfunction, is more common in diabetic male patients. Yet in the SHEP trial, the incidence of sexual dysfunction, as well as symptoms of depression and dementia, were not statistically significantly different between treated and placebo subjects in either nondiabetics or diabetics. In general, adverse effects of therapy were not of great importance in the majority of patients.

Thus both in HDFP, which was a study of diastolic and systolic hypertension in middle-aged individuals, and in SHEP, which was a study of ISH in elderly patients with a mean age of 71, it was apparent that a diuretic-based regimen, with a β-blocker added if necessary, reduced mortality and morbidity due to CHD in diabetic individuals.

In the SHEP study, baseline DBP was <80 mm Hg (mean 77 mm Hg) and reduced by treatment to <75

TABLE 6.3 — Symptoms in Active-Therapy Diabetic Subjects Compared With Placebo Subjects in the Systolic Hypertension in the Elderly Program

Symptom	Diabetics (%)	Nondiabetics (%)
Cold/numb hands		
Active therapy	25	17
Placebo	17	14
Sexual dysfunction		
Active therapy	12	7
Placebo	6	6
Depression		
Active therapy	9	5
Placebo	6	5
Dementia		
Active therapy	2	2
Placebo	2	2

mm Hg in the majority of patients (mean 68 mm Hg) without evidence of a deleterious effect on ischemic heart disease events. There was no evidence to support the concept that lowering DBP to <80-85 mm Hg would increase CHD events. But if DBP was reduced to <55-60 mm Hg, some increase in CHD events was noted. These levels, however, are rarely reached in clinical practice

Thus in these early trials, the benefits of antihypertensive therapy were shown to be as great or even greater in diabetics than in nondiabetic subjects. Thiazide diuretics and β-blockers were used as baseline therapy in these studies as well as in all others prior to the mid 1990s.

In the 1970s and 1980s, it was widely publicized that the use of these agents, especially thiazide diuretics, might actually be dangerous in diabetic patients. The studies reporting this were usually retrospective case report studies with poor follow-up. After the publication of one article that suggested an increase in insulin resistance with diuretics and β-blockers, physicians were advised that these drugs should not be used in diabetics. Other comments that the use of these agents had failed to reduce CHD events while reducing stroke and heart failure also served to indicate to physicians that these were not drugs of choice, especially in diabetic individuals.

A careful review of the early data, however, and the results of more recent trials indicate that not only are thiazide diuretics and β-blockers not harmful, they are clearly beneficial in the management of diabetic hypertensive patients. As noted in SHEP, when diabetic subjects were treated with chlorthalidone initially with atenolol added if goal BP levels were not achieved, outcome was improved. And in the HDFP trial, mortality and morbidity were reduced significantly in the diabetic cohort. In this study, diuretics, β-blockers, hydralazine, and reserpine were the main drugs of choice. Thus physicians who were avoiding the use of these agents were being influenced more by promotional data about newer drugs than by results of carefully controlled, randomized, long-term treatment trials. Recent trials have helped to clarify the role of these as well as other medications in the management of the hypertensive diabetic.

The question of the occurrence of hyperglycemia or new-onset diabetes (NOD) with diuretics and/or β-blockers is discussed in Chapter 7, *Cardiovascular Risk Reduction in Hypertensive Diabetics*. On balance, it does not appear that diuretic use increases NOD by more than about 1% compared with placebo. On the other hand, β-blockers increase NOD to a greater degree and the use of a renin-angiotensin-aldosterone system (RAAS) inhibitor (angiotensin-converting enzyme [ACE] inhibitor or angiotensin II receptor blocker [ARB]) as part of a therapeutic regimen may have a beneficial effect and actually decrease the occurrence of NOD in hypertensive patients compared with regimens that do not include these medications (**Table 5**.**3**).

Therapy for Diabetic Nephropathy

In the 1990s, a series of studies focused on the treatment of diabetic nephropathy, primarily in type 1 diabetes. The main focus of these trials was to determine whether the use of an ACE inhibitor–based treatment program compared with a regimen that did not include an ACE inhibitor would have a beneficial impact on urinary albumin excretion rates as a surrogate of progression of diabetic nephropathy and the occurrence of renal failure. In addition, data on the necessity for dialysis and transplantation were accumulated.

Most of the trials were actually trials of multiple-drug therapy, as were earlier and later studies. For example, in one controlled trial, The Effect of an Angiotensin Converting Enzyme Inhibitor on Diabetic Nephropathy, >75% of patients in the ACE inhibitor group were also receiving thiazide diuretics and β-blockers; these additional medications were necessary to reduce BP to as close to goal as possible. The other treatment group received multiple medications but they did not include an ACE inhibitor. A significant decrease in morbidity/mortality and less progression to renal failure, dialysis, and transplantation were noted in the ACE inhibitor–treated patients (**Table 6**.**4**). There were only minor differences in achieved BP between the two groups. One problem with this trial was that the control group subjects had significantly more proteinuria at baseline (3 g/day) compared with the

TABLE 6.4 — Major Outcome Events in Patients With Type 1 Diabetes and Nephropathy

Event	Number of Patients	
	ACEI + Other Meds	*Other Meds No ACEI*
Death	8	14
Dialysis or transplantation	20	31
Doubling of serum creatinine	23	42
Hyperkalemia	3	0

Abbreviations: ACEI, angiotensin-converting enzyme inhibitors; Meds, medications.

Lewis EJ, et al. *N Engl J Med.* 1993;329:1456.

ACE group (2.5 g/day). Since the degree of proteinuria is predictive of the stage of renal function deterioration, it is possible that the non–ACE-treated group had more renal disease at baseline than the ACE-treated group (**Table 6.5**). This could have affected results.

Similar benefits have been reported when BP was lowered in type 1 diabetics with nephropathy with a combination of thiazide diuretics, β-blockers, and hydralazine. These data indicate that lowering BP with multiple medications, one of which decreases the activity of the RAAS, results in slowing down progression of renal disease (β-blockers decrease the generation of renin; ACE inhibitors block conversion to angiotensin II; and while ARBs do not decrease production of angiotensin II, they block its action at the receptor site).

Subsequent studies within the past 4 years with ACE inhibitors and ARBs have confirmed that either of these agents should be part of the treatment regimen in diabetic nephropathy; that there may be ben-

TABLE 6.5 — Baseline Characteristics of Patients With Diabetic Nephropathy in the Captopril and Placebo Groups

Characteristic	Captopril (n = 207)	Placebo (n = 202)	P Value
Hypertensive (%)	75	74	0.91
On antihypertensive therapy (%)	60	59	0.84
Systolic blood pressure	137	140	0.21
Diastolic blood pressure	85	86	0.47
Serum creatinine (mg/dL)	1.3	1.3	—
24-h urinary protein excretion (mg/d)	2500 ± 2500	3000 ± 2600	0.02*

* Statistically significant difference.

Lewis EJ, et al. *N Engl J Med*. 1993;329:1456.

eficial effects on renal function in diabetics independent of effects on BP. Renovascular resistance is decreased by ACE inhibition; blockade of the RAAS may also improve endothelial dysfunction, the propensity toward early atherogenesis, and smooth muscle hypertrophy, all factors noted in diabetic and hypertensive patients. Some studies with ARBs also suggest that the use of these agents will decrease cardiovascular (CV) morbidity and mortality. The clinical trials with these agents have clearly established their role in the management of type 2 diabetic patients with nephropathy (see Reduction of Endpoints in NIDDM With an Angiotensin II Antagonist, Losartan [RENAAL], Irbesartan in Diabetic Nephropathy Trial [IDNT], and Irbesartan Microalbuminuria Type 2 Diabetes Mellitus in Hypertension Patients trial [IRMA 2] discussions later in this chapter).

■ Appropriate Blood Pressure Control in Diabetes Trial and Fosinopril vs Amlodipine Cardiovascular Event Trial

Effects of different medications have been studied in diabetic hypertensive individuals. In the Appropriate Blood Pressure Control in Diabetes (ABCD) trial and the Fosinopril vs Amlodipine Cardiovascular Event Trial (FACET), the use of an ACE inhibitor, enalapril, was compared with two different long-acting dihydropyridine calcium channel blockers (CCBs), nisoldipine or amlodipine. In both of these studies, the use of an ACE inhibitor–based treatment program in type 2 diabetics produced a better outcome than a CCB–based treatment program (**Table 6.6** and **Table 6.7**). Fewer than 500 patients were followed in each of these trials for approximately 2 to 3 or 5 years. The total number of events was small, especially in FACET.

Blood pressure decreases in the ABCD trial were equal with both classes of drugs, but in FACET, BP decrease was actually greater with amlodipine than

TABLE 6.6 — Adjusted Cardiovascular Events in the Appropriate Blood Pressure Control in Diabetes Study*†

Event	Nisoldipine (n = 235)	Enalapril (n = 235)
Fatal/nonfatal MI	25‡	5‡
Nonfatal MI	22‡	5‡
Cerebrovascular accidents	11	7
Congestive heart failure	6	5
Death from CV event	10	5
Death from any cause	17	13

Abbreviations: CV, cardiovascular; MI, myocardial infarction.

* 93 patients assigned to nisoldipine also needed a diuretic and 89 patients required a β-blocker to achieve goal blood pressure (BP); in the enalapril group, 99 patients required a β-blocker and 110 patients required a diuretic to achieve goal BP.
† 5-year follow-up.
‡ Significant difference between groups.

Adapted from: Estacio RO, et al. *N Engl J Med.* 1998;338:645-652.

with an RAAS inhibitor fosinopril (–19/8 vs –13/8 mm Hg). This has also been noted in other trials such as the recently completed Valsartan Antihypertensive Long-term Use Evaluation (VALUE) trial, where BP lowering was greater with amlodipine (plus other medications) compared with valsartan, an ARB (plus other medications). Despite a similar or lesser degree of BP lowering when compared with the CCB, the ACE inhibitor group in both trials experienced fewer MIs and fewer heart failure episodes. These studies have been criticized for trial design problems and for lack of predictive power (small number of events) but appear to strengthen the argument that ACE inhibitors,

TABLE 6.7 — Cardiovascular Events in the Fosinopril vs Amlodipine Cardiovascular Events Trial*		
Event	Fosinopril (n = 189)	Amlodipine (n = 191)
Fatal/nonfatal stroke	4	5
Fatal/nonfatal MI	10	13
Hospitalized for angina	0	4
Any major CV event	14[†]	27[†]

Abbreviations: CV, cardiovascular; MI, myocardial infarction.

* Mean age of patients 63 years; 3.5-year follow-up.
[†] $P = 0.03$.

Tatti P, et al. *Diabetes Care*. 1998;21:597-603.

usually in combination with a diuretic, are probably to be preferred to CCBs in the management of diabetic nephropathy.

What the FACET and ABCD studies did not suggest was that the use of CCBs in the management of hypertensive diabetic patients is dangerous. For example, *untreated* diabetics in other follow-up studies appeared to experience the same outcome as those treated with CCBs in the ABCD trial. In addition, in FACET, outcome was improved when a CCB was added to the ACE inhibitor. Benefit was greater than with the ACE inhibitor alone. There is a place for the use of CCBs in the treatment of such patients, but it might not be as initial therapy. These studies laid the groundwork for trials that explored specific effects of BP lowering with different medications in diabetic patients *with or without evidence of renal involvement*.

■ The United Kingdom Prospective Diabetes Study

The United Kingdom Prospective Diabetes Study (UKPDS) was a large, prospective, randomized clinical trial that was reported in September 1998. There were several facets of this trial; one was to assess the impact of intense compared with conventional glycemic control on diabetes-related and other end points. The second was to determine the effect of tight BP control compared with less effective BP control on CV events. The third was to evaluate differences in outcome with different antihypertensive regimens.

Four thousand two hundred ninety seven type 2 diabetics were recruited; 1544 were hypertensive and attending hypertension clinics, 421 had previously received treatment but had BP >150/85 mm Hg, and 727 were admitted to the trial as untreated hypertensives with BP >160/90 mm Hg. The mean age was 56 years. The hypertension phase of the study recruited 1148 patients. These patients with type 2 diabetes were randomized to less-tight vs tight BP control groups (**Figure 6.3**). Initial BPs were 160/94 and 159/94 mm Hg, respectively. The tight BP control group was further subdivided into patients randomly assigned to an ACE inhibitor–based regimen (captopril 25 to 50 mg bid) or to a β-blocker–based regimen (atenolol 50 to 100 mg/qd) (**Table 6.8**). Additional drug therapy included the use of furosemide (20 mg daily), a dihydropyridine calcium antagonist (nifedipine SR 10 to 40 mg bid), an α-blocker (prazosin 1 to 5 mg tid), or a centrally acting agent (α-methyldopa 250 to 500 mg bid). Medications other than ACE inhibitors or β-blockers were used in the less-tight control group.

At the end of an 8½-year period, the tight BP control group (297) had achieved BP of 144/82 mm Hg compared with levels of 154/87 mm Hg in the less-tight control group (156). Thus there was a –10/–5 mm Hg difference in achieved BP. Both groups received

FIGURE 6.3 — United Kingdom Prospective Diabetes Study

All randomized patients with type 2 diabetes (n = 4297)

↓

Patients with hypertension, mean age 56 years, mean BP 160/94 mm Hg (n = 1148)

- Less-tight control level achieved 154/87 mm Hg (n = 390)
  - Medications other than ACE inhibitors or β-blockers
- Tight control level achieved 144/82 mm Hg (n = 758)
  - ACE inhibitor–based regimen (n = 400)
  - β-Blocker–based regimen (n = 400)

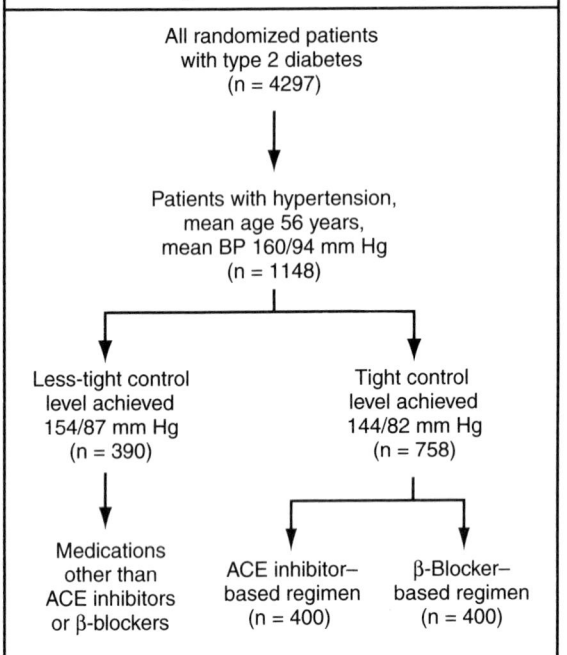

Abbreviations: ACE, angiotensin-converting enzyme; BP, blood pressure.

Difference in achieved BPs: –10/–5 mm Hg; follow-up 8.4 years.

United Kingdom Prospective Diabetes Study Group. *BMJ*. 1998; 317:703-713.

multiple drugs in an attempt to achieve goal BP; about two thirds of the tight control group required two or more different agents; far fewer patients in the less-tight cohort were on two or more drugs. This presumably reflected less of a concerted effort to lower BP. The final results of this 8½-year study are of great interest.

> **TABLE 6.8 — Results of Different Levels of Blood Pressure Control in Hypertensive Patients With Type 2 Diabetes: β-Blocker Compared With ACE Inhibitor–Based Treatment Program**
>
> - Better control of blood pressure (BP) compared with less aggressive treatment in 8.4-year follow-up of 1148 subjects (achieved BP of 144/82 mm Hg compared with 154/87 mm Hg)
> - Reduced risk of:
>   – Stroke (44%)
>   – Fatal strokes (58%)
>   – Death related to diabetes (32%)
>   – Heart failure (56%)
>   – Fatal and nonfatal coronary heart disease events (21%) (trend but not significant)
> - *No difference in outcome between a captopril-based and an atenolol-based treatment program*
>
> Abbreviation: ACE, angiotensin-converting enzyme.
>
> United Kingdom Prospective Diabetes Study Group. *BMJ*. 1998;317:703-713.

A difference of only –10/–5 mm Hg between the two groups of diabetic hypertensives resulted in a reduction of both macrovascular and microvascular events. Reductions of more than 44% in total strokes, 58% in fatal strokes, 21% in MIs, and 56% in heart failure were noted (**Table 6.8**). Of importance is that diabetes-related end points were reduced overall by 24%, diabetes-related deaths by 32%, and microvascular disease (ie, retinopathy progression, loss of visual acuity, and proteinuria) by 37% (**Table 6.9**). Tighter BP control accounted for a dramatic decrease in both microvascular and macrovascular events. Of further interest is the fact that no difference in outcome was noted between the ACE inhibitor–based and the β-blocker–based groups. **Figure 6.4** presents specific data and risk reduction (events/1000 patient years in

TABLE 6.9 — United Kingdom Prospective Diabetes Study: Effect of Blood Pressure Control on Diabetic Events

Tight blood pressure control (144/82 mm Hg) compared with less-effective control (154/87 mm Hg)

Reduction of:
- 24% in diabetic-related end points
- 32% in deaths related to diabetes
- 37% in microvascular events, renal failure, and severe retinopathy

United Kingdom Prospective Diabetes Study Group. *BMJ*. 1998;317:703-713.

the UKPDS trial). While the β-blocker group experienced more side effects and more weight gain than the ACE inhibitor group, the results of this study should help put to rest some of the concerns about using β-blockers in patients with diabetes. It is important to note that the patients receiving β-blockers did not have an increased prevalence of hypoglycemia. Thus the concern about masking the symptoms of low blood glucose levels may only be of clinical relevance in type 1 diabetic patients. Physicians should feel more comfortable about using β-blockers when they may be indicated in diabetic patients, ie, in angina, post MI, or hypertension. Glycemic control in this study was not ideal, as recently defined. HbA_{1C} was 7.2% during the first 4 years and 8.3% over 5 to 8 years. Adequate glycemic control is presently defined as an HbA_{1C} of <7%. No difference in blood glucose control between the ACE inhibitor–based and the β-blocker–based treatment groups was noted.

■ The Captopril Prevention Project Study

Within the past 3 to 4 years, results of several other trials that were based on the use of an ACE inhibitor have been reported. The 5-year ACE inhibitor

Captopril Prevention Project (CAPPP) study, which was a multicenter randomized, prospective, open trial but in which investigators were unaware of the occurrence of end points, included more than 10,000 patients with hypertension and a supine DBP >100 mm Hg. The study compared the ACE inhibitor captopril 50 to 100 mg daily (with hydrochlorothiazide and, in some cases, diltiazem added if necessary), with a regimen of a β-blocker or a diuretic or a combination of both drugs (with diltiazem added, if necessary). There are no data available on the exact number of subjects in the captopril group who required the addition of the thiazide or the number of subjects in the other treatment group who received both a β-blocker and a diuretic, but the percentage of subjects on combined therapy was high.

All-cause mortality and relative risk of CV events were similar in both groups (difference not significant). The occurrence of stroke appeared to be more common in the captopril-based nondiabetic treatment group. However, in the patients with diabetes, the occurrence of MI and all fatal and cardiac events was reduced to a statistically significant greater extent in the captopril-based treatment group compared with the β-blocker–based group (**Figure 6.5** and **Table 6.10**). The incidence of NOD was also significantly lower by 14% in the captopril group. Some differences in baseline characteristics (poor randomization) may explain some of these findings, ie, initial BP was higher in the captopril group (to possibly account for more strokes in these patients), but there was a higher percentage of patients with pretreatment evidence of ischemic heart disease in the β-blocker group (which might account for some of the differences in the CHD event rates in favor of the ACE inhibitor group).

While findings in diabetics are somewhat different in the CAPPP trial than in the UKPDS trial, both

FIGURE 6.4 — Results of Tight Blood Pressure Control Compared With Less-Tight Blood Pressure Control in the United Kingdom Prospective Diabetes Study

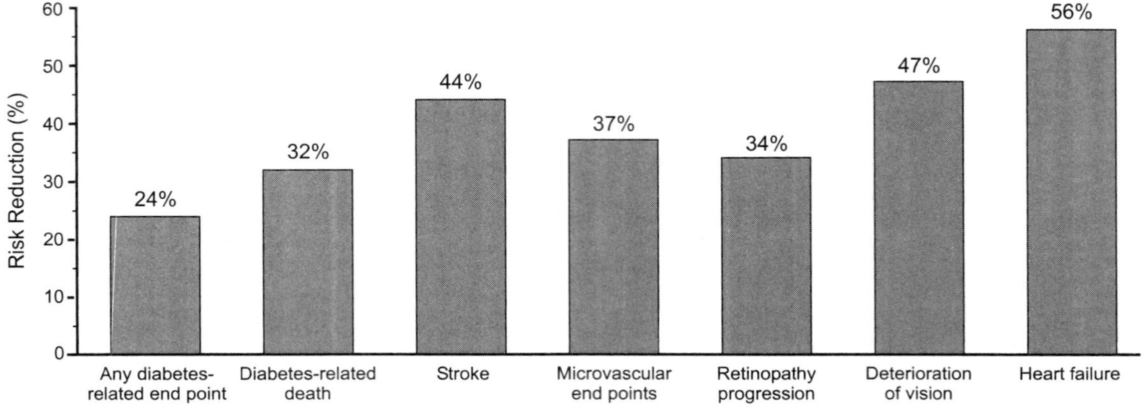

End point	Risk Reduction (%)
Any diabetes-related end point	24%
Diabetes-related death	32%
Stroke	44%
Microvascular end points	37%
Retinopathy progression	34%
Deterioration of vision	47%
Heart failure	56%

Compared with less-tight control, tight control of blood pressure produced a 24% reduction in the risk of diabetes-related mortality, stroke, and microvascular disease ($P = 0.0046$). A combined analysis of all macrovascular diseases (including myocardial infarction, sudden death, stroke, and peripheral vascular disease) showed that tight control was associated with a 34% reduction risk when compared with less-tight control ($P = 0.019$).

All changes are statistically significant.

United Kingdom Prospective Diabetes Study Group. *BMJ*. 1998;317:703-713.

FIGURE 6.5 — Comparison of Captopril–Based and β-Blocker/Diuretic–Based Therapy in Patients With Diabetes in the Captopril Prevention Project (CAPPP)

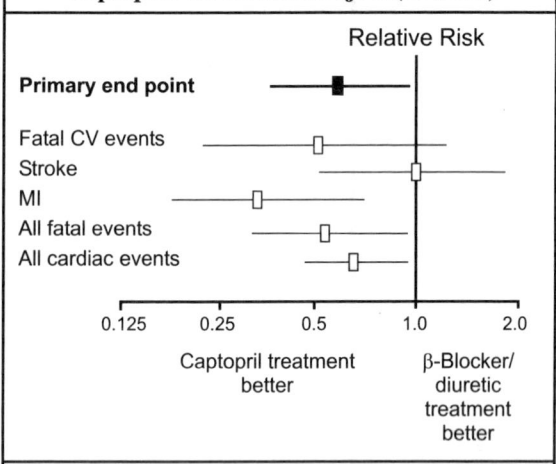

A significant reduction in all cardiovascular (CV) events, myocardial infarctions (MIs), fatal events, and cardiac events was noted in the captopril-based treatment group compared with the β-blocker group in diabetic subjects.

of these studies indicate that in these patients an ACE inhibitor-based treatment program will reduce CV events (except possibly stroke) to as great (or greater) degree as a β-blocker/diuretic–based program. This is consistent with the recommendations of the Sixth and Seventh Joint National Committees (JNCs) on Prevention, Evaluation, Detection, and Treatment of High Blood Pressure that an ACE inhibitor or another RAAS inhibitor should be one component in a treatment program in hypertensive diabetics.

■ Systolic Hypertension Trial in Europe

Other trials have compared the effects of CCBs with placebo or with other antihypertensive medica-

TABLE 6.10 — Risk Reduction in Diabetic Subjects* in the Captopril Prevention Project (CAPPP)

Event	Captopril vs Diuretic or β-Blocker Therapy (% Reduction)	P
Composite end points (fatal and nonfatal strokes and MIs)	50	0.02[†]
Stroke (fatal and nonfatal)	None	0.95
Fatal CV events	50	0.09
MIs (fatal and nonfatal)	70	0.01[†]
All CV events	30	0.03[†]

Abbreviations: CV, cardiovascular; MI, myocardial infarction.

* Number of subjects in study, 572.
[†] Statistically significant difference between the two groups of diabetic patients treated with different medications.

tions and have included some diabetic patients. The Systolic Hypertension Trial in Europe (Syst-Eur) was a large, prospective, randomized, clinical trial designed to test the efficacy of a moderately long-acting dihydropyridine CCB, nitrendipine (not available in the United States), compared with a placebo in elderly patients with ISH and a mean age of approximately 70 years. ISH was defined as SBP >160 mm Hg with a DBP <95 mm Hg. (The definition of ISH, which was being used when the study began, is no longer accepted. The new definition of ISH is a BP ≥140/<90 mm Hg.)

There were >4500 patients randomized to placebo or active treatment, which included nitrendipine (10 to 40 mg/day) with the addition or substitution of enalapril (5 to 20 mg/day) or hydrochlorothiazide (12.5 to 25.0 mg/day) or both. Therapy was titrated to reduce SBP by >10 mm Hg or to <150 mm Hg. Follow-up was about 2 years. The placebo-corrected decrease in BP in 4203 nondiabetic subjects was –10.3/4.5 mm Hg. In this study, there was a reduction of 42% in strokes and 26% in overall cardiac end points in treated compared with placebo subjects. This level of risk reduction is similar to that noted in the SHEP study, which used thiazide diuretics as initial therapy with β-blockers added if necessary.

There were 492 diabetic subjects, about 10% of the total number of patients in the Syst-Eur study. A BP reduction of –8.6/–3.9 mm Hg was noted in the treated diabetic hypertensive patients compared with subjects who received placebo. Overall event rates were reduced significantly in the treated patients compared with placebo subjects (**Table 6.11**). In addition, treatment of hypertension in these subjects was asso-

TABLE 6.11 — Systolic Hypertension in the Elderly Trial*: Results in Diabetics

- Blood pressure changes—difference between therapy and placebo: –9/–4 mm Hg
- In the placebo subjects, the rate of events in diabetics was twice that in nondiabetics. Rate of events became equal in treated diabetics compared with nondiabetics
- Therapy compared with placebo:
  – Reduction of 63% in CV events
  – Reduction of 69% in strokes
  – Reduction of >70% in CV mortality

Abbreviation: CV, cardiovascular.

Absolute benefit was 36 compared with 8 CV events/100 patient years that were prevented in diabetics and nondiabetics, respectively.

* Nitrendipine-based therapy.

ciated with an even greater benefit in terms of CVD risk reduction than that observed in nondiabetic patients. For example, in diabetic patients, there was a 55% reduction in total mortality compared with a 6% reduction in nondiabetics, a >70% reduction in CV mortality compared with a 13% reduction in nondiabetics, and a 69% reduction in fatal and nonfatal strokes compared with 38% in nondiabetics. All cardiac events combined were reduced by 53% compared with 26% in nondiabetics. The study concluded that the excess CVD risk and mortality usually associated with diabetics compared with nondiabetics in this elderly population was almost completely abolished by the treatment of hypertension. In this study, unlike the others previously reported, the benefit was based on the use of a longer-acting CCB as initial or baseline therapy.

It may seem counterintuitive that risk is reduced to a greater degree in diabetic hypertensive patients than in nondiabetics, but it is well known that the greater the risk and the greater the number of risk factors, the better the results of therapy. Simply stated, benefit is greatest in patients at high risk or in the elderly (who usually are at high risk with multiple risk factors). This was noted in the SHEP and UKPDS studies. Another major multidrug trial that used a CCB as baseline therapy (Hypertension Optimal Treatment [HOT] trial) appeared to confirm that BP should be set lower in diabetic patients.

■ Hypertension Optimal Treatment Trial

The HOT study was designed to determine the optimal target BP that would result in the lowest morbidity/mortality that could be achieved in treated hypertensive patients. More than 18,000 patients from 26 European countries were randomly assigned to one of three target BP groups, <90, <85, or <80 mm Hg DBP. There were no target BP levels set for SBP. In this trial as in others, with the exception of the ISH studies (SHEP and Syst-Eur), goal BP was established only for DBP.

In recent years, it has become apparent that elevated SBP is a more accurate indicator of CV risk than DBP. For example, while most physicians will treat a patient with a persistent DBP of 95 to 100 mm Hg, many will not treat a patient with a SBP of 150 to 159 mm Hg and a normal DBP; yet, SBP at these levels poses a greater risk for CV events than DBP of 95 to 100 mm Hg (**Figure 6.6**). This may be especially true in diabetic subjects where many of the patients with type 2 diabetes are >60 years of age and have predominantly SBP elevations. Yet, as was the custom with other trials, the HOT study primarily focused on DBP. Changes in SBP were noted and considered in

FIGURE 6.6 — Relative Risk of Elevated Systolic and Diastolic Blood Pressure

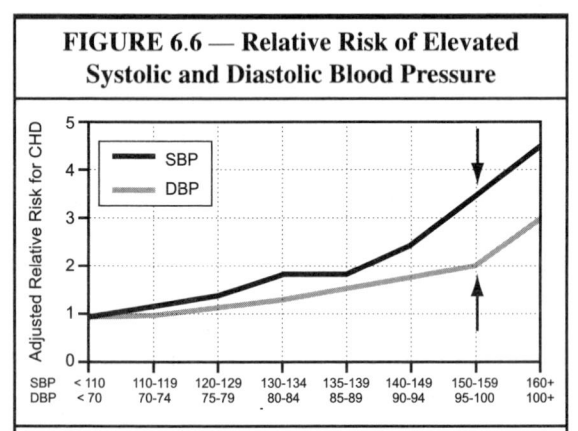

Elevated systolic blood pressure (SBP) may impart greater risk for coronary heart disease (CHD) than elevated diastolic blood pressure (DBP); ie, 150-159 mm Hg SBP poses a greater risk than 95-100 mm Hg DBP. See text.

Data from: Multiple Risk Factor Intervention Trial Research Group. *JAMA*. 1990;263:1795-1801.

the final analysis of events, but these were not considered to be primary considerations.

In the HOT trial, DBP levels were titrated using the dihydropyridine CCB felodipine as primary therapy, with other drugs added as necessary; these included ACE inhibitors, β-blockers, and thiazide diuretics. In many cases, three or more medications were necessary to achieve goal BP. One of the reasons for this may have been that diuretics were only added after the other drugs had been titrated upward. It is quite possible that more subjects would have responded to fewer medications if a diuretic had been added as a second step. Patients were followed for approximately 4 years and the impact of different levels of achieved BP on CV events was recorded. The lowest incidence of major CV events occurred with a mean SBP of 139 mm Hg and a DBP of 83 mm Hg. Lowest CV mortality was noted at levels of 139/87 mm Hg. Most of the benefit therefore occurred in patients who achieved BP <140/90 mm Hg, a level consistent with the recommendations of most US and international guidelines for a majority of hypertensive individuals.

Within the HOT study, there were 1501 (8%) diabetic subjects. Among all of the patients in the HOT trial, there was little difference in overall morbidity/mortality between those who achieved <90 mm Hg, <85 mm Hg, or <80 mm Hg DBP (actual achieved BP in the three target groups were 85, 83, and 81 mm Hg) (**Figure 6.7**). However, within the diabetic group, there was a significant difference between groups. There was a 51% reduction in CV events and a reduction of 43% in CV mortality in hypertensive diabetic patients who achieved target BP of ≤80 mm Hg compared with those in the <90 mm Hg cohort (**Figure 6.8**). Targets achieved were 140/81 mm Hg compared with 144/85 mm Hg, a difference of only –4/–4 mm Hg. Thus this trial, as well as the MD Renal Disease and the UKPDS

FIGURE 6.7 — Patients With Diabetes in the Hypertension Optimal Treatment Trial

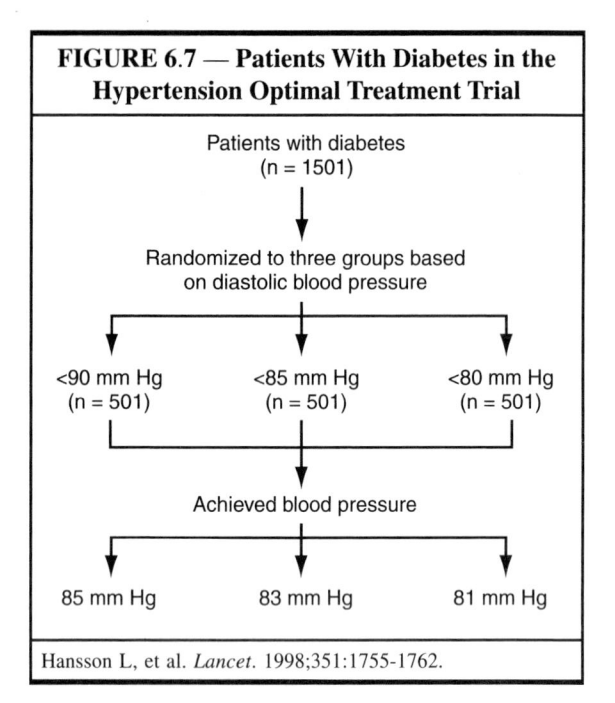

Patients with diabetes (n = 1501)
↓
Randomized to three groups based on diastolic blood pressure

| <90 mm Hg (n = 501) | <85 mm Hg (n = 501) | <80 mm Hg (n = 501) |

↓
Achieved blood pressure

| 85 mm Hg | 83 mm Hg | 81 mm Hg |

Hansson L, et al. *Lancet*. 1998;351:1755-1762.

trials, indicates that targeting lower BP in diabetics than in nondiabetics is beneficial. These observations are consistent with the idea that diabetic subjects have an increased tendency toward vascular injury when BP is even slightly elevated and that reducing BP to as close to the normotensive range or ideal BP of 120/80 mm Hg is a goal to be achieved if at all possible. Again, the JNCs, the National Kidney Foundation, and the American Diabetes Association recommendations for lower BP goals in diabetics seem reasonable.

In the HOT trial, the use of aspirin proved beneficial in reducing coronary heart disease events in diabetic patients as well as in the rest of the study population. There appears to be little danger and potential benefit of aspirin therapy in hypertensive subjects *if their BP is controlled.*

FIGURE 6.8 — Cardiovascular Events in Diabetics in the Hypertension Optimal Treatment Study

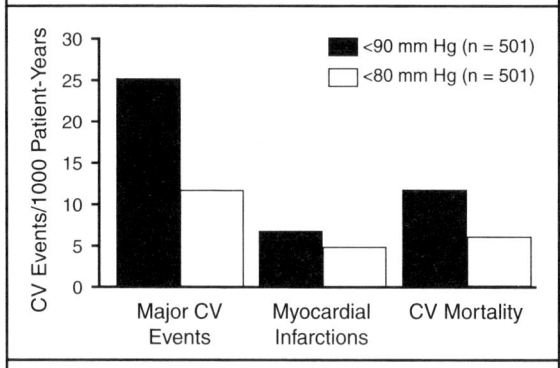

Cardiovascular (CV) events were reduced to a greater degree in diabetics who achieved the lowest levels of diastolic blood pressure.

Hansson L, et al. *Lancet*. 1998;351:1755-1762.

The HOT study, as well as the UKPDS, pointed out the need to rethink our approach to the diabetic patient and to emphasize that management of hypertension may be as or more important than glycemic control in these patients. Thus the emphasis should shift from glycemic control *alone* to a more multifaceted approach. There was no evidence in the diabetic cohort in the HOT study, or in other trials such as UKPDS or Syst-Eur, to suggest that aggressive treatment is harmful or that it increases MI or ischemic heart disease events. Although the concept of the J-curve is an interesting one (ie, that reducing DBP <80-85 mm Hg might actually increase the number of ischemic heart disease events in patients with plaque formation or previous ischemic heart disease), there is little evidence that there may be an adverse effect before DBP levels decrease to <55-60 mm Hg. As noted, these lower levels are infrequently achieved in clinical practice.

Both the HOT and the SHEP studies strongly suggest that decreasing DBP to <80 mm Hg is not only safe but may actually decrease the number of ischemic heart disease events. In fact, the lower the better in diabetics, consistent with a lack of adverse effects. Many physicians are concerned about treating the elderly diabetic patient because of fear of decreasing DBP too much in these patients who primarily have ISH. Again, the HOT study, as well as others, seems to have put that fear to rest. Many diabetics >65 years of age will have BP of 150-180/80-85 mm Hg. Decreasing the SBP to more normal levels is clearly beneficial, even if the DBP decreases to levels of 70-75 mm Hg.

It is important to note that *most of the medications that are currently in use decrease SBP to a greater degree than DBP and reduce pulse pressure*. An increased pulse pressure is indicative of increased vascular rigidity, an important prognostic indicator of increased risk. There are no data yet to indicate that decreasing pulse pressure improves prognosis, but a decrease may indicate some decrease in vessel rigidity that may be beneficial. There is no reason why a patient with or without diabetes with elevated SBP with normal DBP should not have their BP reduced.

The well-controlled, randomized clinical trials, which now have included >7,000 diabetic hypertensive patients, have clearly indicated that lowering BP is beneficial; morbidity and mortality, not just from macrovascular but also from microvascular events, will be reduced. All of the clinical trials in diabetic patients reported to date indicate that in a majority of cases, it is possible to reduce BP to goal levels or near goal levels of 130/80-85 mm Hg with the available antihypertensive medications with or without lifestyle interventions. It is obvious from these trials that often more than one medication is required. In fact, in diabetic patients, there is some evidence to suggest that the use of a combination of drugs as initial therapy, eg, an ACE inhibitor and a diuretic, an ARB/diuretic combination, or in some instances, a β-blocker/diuretic combination, might be appropriate.

What Role Do the ARBs Have in the Management of Diabetic Patients?

■ RENAAL, IDNT, and IRMA 2 Studies

The results of three other trials, RENAAL, IDNT, and IRMA 2 have helped to clarify the role of ARBs in the management of the diabetic patient with varying degrees of renal disease. Both of these last two trials were part of the Program for Irbesartan Morbidity and Mortality Evaluation (PRIME) research program.

RENAAL

RENAAL was a 3-year, multinational controlled trial evaluating the effects on renal function of an ARB, losartan (Cozaar) 50-100 mg/day, when added to other medications in 1513 type 2 diabetic patients. The group on losartan was compared with similar patients whose therapy included antihypertensive medications other than an ACE inhibitor or an ARB (the "placebo" group). Patients had average baseline BP of 153/82 mm Hg with evidence of diabetic nephropathy with proteinuria (>500 mg/day) and mean baseline creatinine levels of 1.9 mg/dL. At the end of the trial, there was a significant reduction in the risk of renal disease progression with fewer patients requiring renal dialysis or transplantation in the ARB group compared with the non–ARB-treated group. This was the first study to specifically demonstrate a statistically significant decrease in progression to end-stage renal disease (ESRD) in patients with type 2 diabetic nephropathy. A 16% reduction in the composite end point, doubling of serum creatinine, ESRD, and death was noted. A 28% ($P = 0.002$) decrease in the occurrence of ESRD was noted in the group of patients treated with losartan (**Figure 6.9**). Studies with ACE inhibitor–based therapy had previously reported a reduction in progression of proteinuria in these patients but not a signifi-

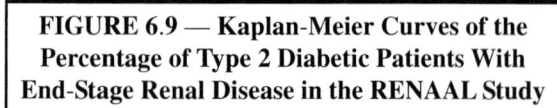

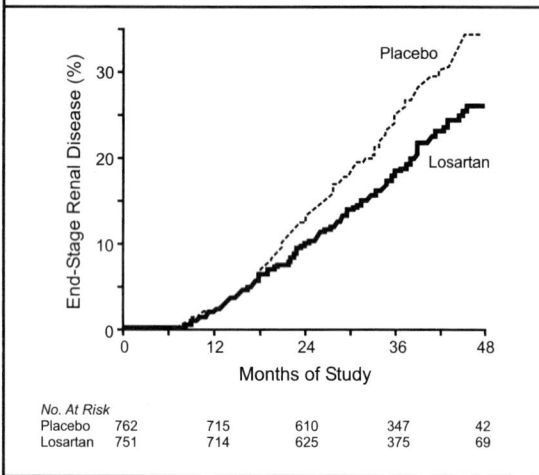

FIGURE 6.9 — Kaplan-Meier Curves of the Percentage of Type 2 Diabetic Patients With End-Stage Renal Disease in the RENAAL Study

No. At Risk					
Placebo	762	715	610	347	42
Losartan	751	714	625	375	69

Abbreviations: ACE, angiotensin-converting enzyme; ARB, angiotensin II receptor blocker; RENAAL, Reduction in Endpoints in Patients NIDDM With the Angiotensin II Antagonist Losartan [study].

Losartan graph line indicates therapy with ARB or other medications, while the placebo line shows therapy with medications other than an ARB or ACE inhibitor. (Risk reduction, 28%; $P = 0.002$.)

* Medications other than an ACE inhibitor or ARB

† Losartan plus other medications

Brenner BM, et al. *N Engl J Med*. 2001;345:865.

cant reduction in ESRD. No difference in mortality or the total number of CV events (a secondary end point) was noted, but 32% ($P = 0.005$) fewer episodes of hospitalization for congestive heart failure occurred in the group receiving the ARB compared with patients who were treated with other agents.

IDNT

IDNT compared results of treatment of three groups of subjects with type 2 diabetes, significant proteinuria, and evidence of renal functional impairment. One thousand seven hundred fifteen patients were randomized to receive 1) an ARB, irbesartan (Avapro), up to 300 mg/qd, in addition to medications other than an ACE inhibitor or a CCB; or 2) amlodipine 2.5-10 mg/qd in addition to other medications other than the study drugs; or 3) medications other than the study drugs (a so-called placebo group).

Mean duration of the study was 2.6 years. Primary end point of the study was a composite end point of development of ESRD, death from any cause, and the time to doubling of the serum creatinine concentration (**Figure 6.10**). Treatment with irbesartan plus other medications that did not include an ACE inhibitor, another ARB, or a CCB resulted in a significant 20% reduction in risk of the primary end point and 33% reduction in the risk of doubling of serum creatinine compared with patients treated with medications other than an ACE inhibitor, ARB, or CCB ("placebo" group). Of interest was the finding of a 23% reduction ($P = 0.006$) in the primary end point and a 37% reduction ($P = 0.001$) in risk of doubling of creatinine in the irbesartan group compared with subjects on a regimen based on amlodipine (plus other medications except ARBs and ACE inhibitors). Achieved BP differences between the ARB and CCB group were not significant. Proteinuria was also significantly reduced

FIGURE 6.10 — Cumulative Proportions of Patients Reaching Primary End Points* in the IDNT

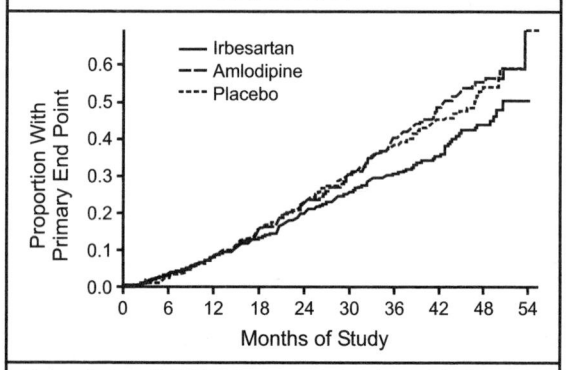

Abbreviation: IDNT, Irbesartan in Diabetic Nephropathy Trial.

Proportion of patients with primary end points. Differences between irbesartan and placebo and irbesartan and amlodipine were significant (–20% [$P = 0.02$] and –23% [$P = 0.006$], respectively).

* Doubling of baseline serum creatinine, end-stage renal disease, and death from any cause.

Lewis EJ, et al. *N Engl J Med.* 2001;345:856.

in the irbesartan group compared with other therapies. No difference in all-cause mortality was noted among groups in this trial. This trial provides some additional evidence to suggest a better outcome in patients with diabetes and renal disease who are treated with a RAAS inhibitor compared with those on a CCB.

IRMA 2

The IRMA 2 trial compared the effects on patients of irbesartan (150 or 300 mg/day) plus other medications (other than ACE inhibitors or ARBs) with patients on medications other than an ARB or ACE inhibitor.

Five hundred ninety type 2 diabetic patients who demonstrated microproteinuria (30-300 mg/day) were followed for 2 years. No significant differences in achieved BP were noted in the three groups of patients. There was, however, a 70% reduction in progression to more severe renal disease in the group of patients treated with irbesartan; doses of 300 mg proved to be more effective than the 150-mg dose. The group that received irbesartan 300 mg/day compared with the non-ARB group experienced a significant reduction in the number who progressed to frank proteinuria (>300 mg/day). In addition, 34% normalized the amount of albumin excreted (**Figure 6.11**).

Overview of Completed Trials

In all three of the above trials, the ARB used was well tolerated. The results of these studies have important treatment implications and suggest that recommendations for treatment of hypertension in type 2 diabetics (which previously included the use of ACE inhibitors as a preferred treatment) now include the use of ARBs as well, especially in diabetic nephropathy. As previously noted, one of the trials (IDNT) indicated that renal disease progression can be delayed to a greater extent with an ARB than with a CCB-based treatment program. In all cases, however, multiple medications will usually be necessary to achieve goal BP—treatment should include the use of a diuretic.

Data indicate that not only the progression to more severe renal disease can be slowed by the use of an ARB, but that signs of glomerular dysfunction, ie, proteinuria, may be improved with a decrease in microproteinuria. These findings are similar to those regarding left ventricular hypertrophy (LVH) in hypertension. LVH can be regressed with treatment or actually prevented if BP is lowered in hypertensive individuals before LVH becomes apparent.

FIGURE 6.11 — Progression of Diabetic Nephropathy in IRMA 2 Study of Hypertensive Patients With Type 2 Diabetes and Microproteinuria

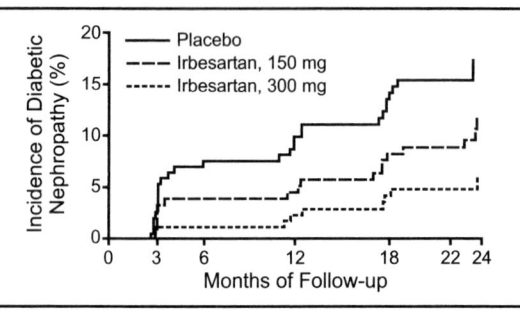

Abbreviations: ACE, angiotensin-converting enzyme; ARB, angiotensin II receptor blocker; IRMA 2, Irbesartan Microalbuminuria Type 2 [study].

Progression of diabetic nephropathy in IRMA 2 study of hypertensive patients with type 2 diabetes and microproteinuria. Placebo represents medications other than an ARB or ACE inhibitor. In the irbesartan 150-mg and 300-mg groups, a medication other than another ARB or ACE inhibitor can be given. The difference between placebo and 150 mg irbesartan was not significant ($P = 0.08$); between placebo and 300 mg irbesartan, $P < 0.001$.

Parving HH, et al. *N Engl J Med*. 2001;345:875.

■ Losartan Intervention for Endpoint Reduction in Hypertension Study

The Losartan Intervention For Endpoint Reduction in Hypertension Study (LIFE) demonstrated a significant reduction in strokes and in the development of diabetes in a group of hypertensive patients with LVH who were treated with an ARB-based (losartan) regimen when compared with patients on a β-blocker–based (atenolol) program (see Chapter 5, *The Renin-Angiotensin-Aldosterone System in Diabetes*, and Chapter 7, *Cardiovascular Risk Reduction in Hyper-*

tensive Diabetics, for differences in NOD between groups). In addition, in a diabetic subgroup treated with ARB therapy, CV events were reduced to a greater extent than in nondiabetics (**Figure 6.12**).

■ Heart Outcome Prevention Evaluation Study

One additional study that included a large number of diabetic subjects is the Heart Outcome Prevention Evaluation (HOPE) study. This was not primarily a trial of patients with hypertension since the average BP prior to entering the trial was 139/79 mm Hg. In this trial, 3577 high-risk patients with diabetes with a mean age >55 years were included. A large majority had multiple risk factors or evidence of ischemic heart disease. Most patients were on multiple drugs for either hypertension or other diseases prior to entering the trial. No patients with clinical proteinuria, heart failure, or low ejection fraction or patients who were taking ACE inhibitors were included in the study. Patients, most of whom were already on multiple medications, were randomly assigned an ACE inhibitor (ramipril 10 mg/day) or placebo. The study was stopped 6 months prematurely after 4 to 5 years because of a consistent benefit in the ACE-inhibitor group compared with the control subjects who were not receiving an ACE inhibitor. The risk of the combined primary outcome was reduced by 25%, MI by 22%, stroke by 33%, CV death by 37%, total mortality by 27%, revascularization by 17%, and overt nephropathy by 24% in the group that received the ACE inhibitor (**Table 6.12**). Primary outcome events were reduced by 25% after adjusting for the changes in SBP and DBP. These were minimal; BP in the ACE group were only 2-4/1 mm Hg lower than in the other group. The CV benefit appeared to be greater than that attributable to the slight decrease in BP. Thus although some of the benefits might be attributable to the changes in BP, it was suggested that in this high-risk

FIGURE 6.12 — Clinical Outcomes Among Diabetic Hypertensives Treated With Losartan or Atenolol in the LIFE Study

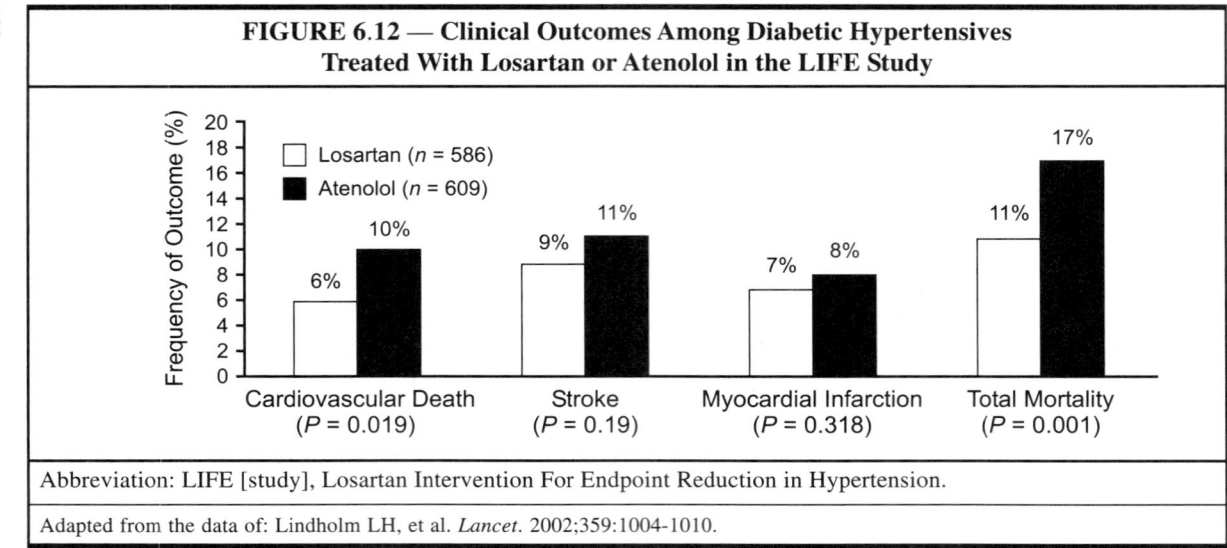

Outcome	Losartan (n = 586)	Atenolol (n = 609)	P value
Cardiovascular Death	6%	10%	0.019
Stroke	9%	11%	0.19
Myocardial Infarction	7%	8%	0.318
Total Mortality	11%	17%	0.001

Abbreviation: LIFE [study], Losartan Intervention For Endpoint Reduction in Hypertension.

Adapted from the data of: Lindholm LH, et al. *Lancet*. 2002;359:1004-1010.

TABLE 6.12 — Results of the Heart Outcome Prevention Evaluation Study in Diabetes*

Event	Reduction in Risk[†]
Combined primary outcome	↓ 25%
Myocardial infarction	↓ 22%
Stroke	↓ 33%
Cardiovascular death	↓ 37%
Total mortality	↓ 27%
Overt nephropathy	↓ 24%

* Number of patients studied 3577, age >55 years.
† Angiotensin-converting enzyme (ACE) inhibitor group compared with subjects not receiving an ACE inhibitor. The use of this agent in addition to other medications reduced cardiovascular events.

group of diabetic patients, the benefit of treatment may have resulted from specific effects of blockade of the RAAS.

As noted in Chapter 5, *The Renin-Angiotensin-Aldosterone System in Diabetes*, blockade of the RAAS has proved to be useful in diabetic patients, not just in improving nephropathy but in reducing some of the basic physiologic changes that are noted in the diabetic—specifically, endothelial dysfunction which is the hallmark of the atherosclerotic process. The HOPE study, therefore, suggests that in high-risk diabetic patients, even in the absence of significant elevations of BP, the use of an ACE inhibitor as part of the program may not only be beneficial in reducing nephropathy complications but in reducing other events. Additional studies are under way to determine whether the use of an ARB when added to other therapies will result in similar levels of CVD event reduction.

A summary of hypertension treatment trials in diabetic patients is provided in **Table 6.13**. It is impor-

TABLE 6.13 — Randomized Controlled Clinical Trials of Antihypertensive Therapy in Type 2 Diabetic Patients With Hypertension

Trial	N	Treatment	F/U (y)	BP Decrease SBP/DPB (mm Hg)	End Points	Risk Reduction: Therapy vs Control (%)
Comparative Trials						
ABCD	470	Nisoldipine Enalapril	2	−20/10 −20/10 (estimated from graph)	Death from CV events	Enalapril vs nisoldipine: −51
CAPPP	632	Captopril + diuretic or CCB β-Blocker or thiazide ± CCB	6	−10/10 (estimated from graph)	Fatal or nonfatal MI; all CV events	Captopril vs conventional therapy: MIs: −66 CV events: −33
FACET	380	Fosinopril (n = 189) Amlodipine (n = 191)	3.5	13/8 19/8	Combined MI, stroke, or hospitalized angina	Fosinopril vs amlodipine: −51
MIDAS	415	Isradipine HCTZ	3	18/13 19/13	CVD events	Isradipine (5.65) vs HCTZ (3.17)

Isolated Systolic Hypertension Trials					
SHEP	583	Chlorthalidone + atenolol or reserpine Placebo	5	Active vs placebo: −9.6/−2.2	Major CVD events Major CHD events Nonfatal MI, fatal CHD Strokes	34 56 54 22
Syst-Eur	492	Nitrendipine + enalapril or HCTZ (n = 252) Placebo (n = 240)	2	Active vs placebo: 10.1/−4.5	CVD mortality CVD events Strokes	76 63 73
Tight Blood Pressure Control vs Less-Tight Control					
HOT	1501	Felodipine + ACEI + β-blocker + diuretic: DBP <90 DBP <85 DBP <80	4–5	 −26.2/20.3 28.0/22.3 29.3/24.3	<90 mm Hg vs <80 mm Hg risk increase (with higher pressure): Major CVD events CVD mortality Total mortality	 +100 +200 +77
UKPDS*	1148	Tight BP control vs less-tight control (n = 390)	8	−10/−5	Diabetes-related end points Diabetes-related deaths Strokes Microvascular	−24 −32 −44 −37

Continued

Trial	N	Treatment	F/U (y)	BP Decrease SBP/DPB (mm Hg)	End Points	Risk Reduction: Therapy vs Control (%)
UKPDS* *(continued)*	1148	β-Blocker (n = 358) vs ACEI program (n = 400)			No significant difference between treatment groups

Abbreviations: ABCD, Appropriate Blood Pressure Control in Diabetes; ACEI, angiotensin-converting enzyme inhibitor; BP, blood pressure; CAPPP, Captopril Prevention Project; CCB, calcium channel blocker; CHD, coronary heart disease; CV, cardiovascular; CVD, cardiovascular disease; DBP, diastolic blood pressure; FACET, Fosinopril vs Amlodipine Cardiovascular Event Trial; F/U, follow-up; HCTZ, hydrochlorothiazide; HOT, Hypertension Optimal Treatment; MI, myocardial infarction; MIDAS, Myocardial Infarction Data Acquisition System analysis; n/N, number [of diabetic subjects in study]; SHEP, Systolic Hypertension in the Elderly Program; Syst-Eur, Systolic Hypertension Trial in Europe; UKPDS, United Kingdom Prospective Diabetes Study.

Trials strongly suggest that strict control of BP in diabetics is beneficial and that a medication that decreases the activity of the renin-aldosterone-angiotensin system should be part of the treatment regimen.

* Number to treat to prevent one event: 15.

Modified from: Chowdhury TA, et al. *J Hum Hypertens*. 1999;13:803-811.

tant to note that there is a trend favoring the use of ACE inhibitor/diuretic therapy, β-blocker/diuretic therapy or, based on recent data, a regimen with an ARB compared with CCB therapy. CCBs can be used in addition to other therapy to lower BP in difficult-to-manage cases. It is also clear that better BP control results in better outcome. Outcome is improved in both young and older diabetics to a great or greater degree than in nondiabetics. These trials have answered many questions that were posed several years ago before the trials were completed (**Table 6.14**). There are now enough data available to indicate vigorous treatment of diabetic patients with hypertension.

SELECTED READING

Brenner BM, Cooper ME, de Zeeuw, et al for the RENAAL Study Investigators. Effects of losartan on renal and cardiovascular outcomes in patients with type 2 diabetes and nephropathy. *N Engl J Med*. 2001;345:861-869.

Chowdhury TA, Kumar S, Barnett AH, Dodson PM. Treatment of hypertension in patients with type 2 diabetes: a review of the recent evidence. *J Hum Hypertens*. 1999;13:803-811.

Curb JD, Pressel SL, Cutler JA, et al. Effect of diuretic-based antihypertensive treatment on cardiovascular disease risk in older diabetic patients with isolated systolic hypertension. Systolic Hypertension in the Elderly Program Cooperative Research Group. *JAMA*. 1996;276:1886-1892.

Estacio RO, Jeffers BW, Hiatt WR, Biggerstaff SL, Gifford N, Schrier RW. The effect of nisoldipine as compared with enalapril on cardiovascular outcomes in patients with non–insulin-dependent diabetes and hypertension. *N Engl J Med*. 1998;338:645-652.

Hansson L, Lindholm LH, Ekborn T, et al. Randomized trial of old and new antihypertensive drugs in elderly patients. Cardiovascular morbidity and mortality in the Swedish Trial in Older Patients with Hypertension-2 study. *Lancet*. 1999;354:1751-1756.

TABLE 6.14 — Answers Provided by the Treatment Trials in Diabetics With Hypertension

- Lowering blood pressure (BP) in hypertensive diabetics reduces cardiovascular (CV) morbidity and mortality: risk reduction is greater than in nondiabetics.
- Lowering BP may be more effective than improving glycemic control.
- Lowering BP will also delay progression of retinopathy and nephropathy.
- Patients should be treated if BP is >140/90 mm Hg.
- Goal for treated BP should be set at ≤130/80-85 mm Hg.
- Treatment programs based on angiotensin-converting enzyme (ACE) inhibitors, angiotensin receptor blockers (ARBs), diuretics, β-blockers, and calcium channel blockers have produced beneficial results; the use of an ACE inhibitor may be more effective in reducing CV events than a calcium channel blocker, especially in patients with nephropathy.
- A treatment regimen that includes an ARB compared with a program without an ARB or ACE inhibitor significantly reduces progression of renal disease in patients with type 2 diabetes.
- Most hypertensive diabetics will require multiple medications to achieve goal BP; therapy should include an ACE inhibitor or an ARB and a diuretic.

Hansson L, Zanchetti A, Carruthers SG, et al. Effects of intensive blood-pressure lowering and low-dose aspirin in patients with hypertension: principal results of the Hypertension Optimal Treatment (HOT) randomised trial. HOT Study Group. *Lancet*. 1998;351:1755-1762.

Lewis EJ, Hunsicker LG, Bain RP, Rohde RD. The effect of angiotensin-converting-enzyme inhibition on diabetic nephropathy. The Collaborative Study Group [published erratum appears in *N Engl J Med*. 1993;330:152]. *N Engl J Med*. 1993;329:1456-1462.

Lewis EJ, Hunsicker LG, Clarke WR, et al. Renoprotective effect of the angiotensin-receptor antagonist irbesartan in patients with nephropathy due to type 2 diabetes. *N Engl J Med*. 2001;345:851-860.

Lindholm LH, Ibsen H, Dahlof, B, et al for the LIFE Study Group. Cardiovascular morbidity and mortality in patients with diabetes in the Losartan Intervention for Endpoint Reduction in Hypertension study (LIFE): a randomised trial against atenolol. *Lancet*. 2002;359:1004-1010.

McInnes GT, Yeo WW, Ramsay L, Moser M. Cardiotoxicity and diuretics: much speculation—little substance. *J Hypertens*. 1992;10:317-335. Editorial.

Moser M. Current hypertension management, separating fact from fiction. *Cleve Clin J Med*. 1993;60:27-37.

Moser M. Is it time for a new approach to the initial treatment of hypertension? *Arch Intern Med*. 2001;161:1040-1045.

Moser M, Hebert PR. Prevention of disease progression, left ventricular hypertrophy and congestive heart failure in the hypertension treatment trials. *J Am Coll Cardiol*. 1996;27:1214-1218.

Multiple Risk Factor Intervention Trial Research Group. Mortality rates after 10.5 years for participants in the Multiple Risk Factor Intervention Trial. Findings related to a priori hypotheses of the trial. *JAMA*. 1990;263:1795-1801.

Parving HH, Lehnert H, Brochner-Mortensen J, Gomis R, Andersen S, Arner P. The effect of irbesartan on the development of diabetic nephropathy in patients with type 2 diabetes. *N Engl J Med*. 2001;345:870-878.

SHEP Investigators. Prevention of stroke by antihypertensive drug treatment in older person with isolated systolic hypertension: final results of the Systolic Hypertension in the Elderly Program (SHEP). *JAMA*. 1991;265:3255-3264.

Sowers JR. Treatment of hypertension in patients with diabetes. *Arch Intern Med*. 2004;164:1850-1857.

Staessen JA, Fagard R, Thijis L, et al for the Systolic Hypertension Europe (Syst-Eur) Trial Investigators. Morbidity and mortality in the placebo-controlled European Trial on Isolated Systolic Hypertension in the Elderly. *Lancet*. 1997;350:757-764.

Tatti P, Pahor M, Byington RP, et al. Outcome results of the Fosinopril Versus Amlodipine Cardiovascular Events Randomized Trial (FACET) in patients with hypertension and NIDDM. *Diabetes Care*. 1998;21:597-603.

United Kingdom Prospective Diabetes Study Group. Tight blood pressure control and risk of macrovascular and microvascular complications in type 2 diabetes: UKPDS 38. UK Prospective Diabetes Study Group. *BMJ*. 1998;317:703-713.

7 Cardiovascular Risk Reduction in Hypertensive Diabetics

General Approach

Tight blood pressure (BP) control has been shown to be an important strategy in reducing both macrovascular and microvascular disease in patients with diabetes mellitus. The target goal for treatment of hypertension in this high-risk population has been set at either 130/85 or 130/80 mm Hg, depending on the organization recommending specific therapy (**Figure 7.1**).

There are a number of unique challenges in adequately treating hypertension in this population. First, many of these patients are overweight and care must be taken in choosing the appropriate-sized cuff so as to avoid errors in BP measurement. Use of a standard-sized BP cuff in an obese patient will often lead to an overestimation of BP levels. This may lead to an inappropriate diagnosis of hypertension. A larger sized cuff should be used in such patients.

Second, BP in diabetics is often more labile, especially systolic blood pressure (SBP), than in the general population. This often necessitates more measurements over a longer time period to adequately assess the casual BP. In addition, many persons with diabetes are nondippers and lose the normal drop of about 10% in nocturnal BP, which likely reflects both autonomic dysfunction and/or abnormal renal sensing of supine changes in volume/perfusion pressure (responsiveness of the autonomic nervous system is blunted). This "nondipping" property of BP at night suggests that the office BP measurement may underpredict the

FIGURE 7.1 — Suggested Treatment Program for Patients With Hypertension and Type 2 Diabetes

Blood pressure >140/90 mm Hg
↓

Lifestyle interventions:
- Especially weight loss, if appropriate
- Sodium restriction
- Moderate exercise

Plus

Antihypertensive medications

↓ ↓

*Preferred Therapy**
ACE inhibitor or ARB, usually with a diuretic

Alternate Therapy[†]
β-Blocker with a diiuretic

↓

Goal blood pressure of >130-135/80-85 mm Hg not achieved

↓ ↓

Add a CCB or β-blocker

Add an ACE inhibitor or ARB

↓

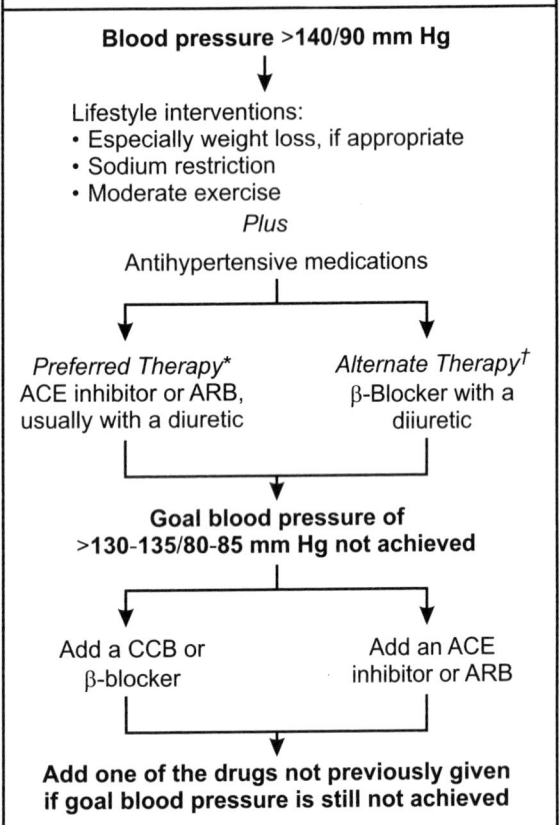

Add one of the drugs not previously given if goal blood pressure is still not achieved

Abbreviations: ACE, angiotensin-converting enzyme; ARB, angiotensin II receptor blocker; CCB, calcium channel blocker; HCTZ, hydrochlorothiazide.

* Medications that might be used include an ACE inhibitor (ie, ramipril, accupril, or lisinopril) as monotherapy in dosages from 5 to 20 mg once daily, or in a combination with a diuretic, such as Vaseretic or Zestoretic, each of which contains 12.5 mg HCTZ. An ARB might

> be any one listed in **Table 7.9**, ie, losartan (Cozaar) 50 mg titrated up to 100 mg/day, irbesartan (Avapro) 150-300 mg, candesartan (Atacand) 16 mg titrated to 32 mg, or valsartan (Diovan) 80-160 mg, or combinations of these medications, such as Hyzaar (with 12.5 mg of HCTZ), Avalide (with 12.5 mg of HCTZ), Atacand HCT (with 12.5 mg of HCTZ), or Diovan HCT (with 12.5 mg of HCTZ).
> † Ziac (a combination of the β-blocker bisoprolol 2.5 or 5 mg and a diuretic 6.25 mg HCTZ) or Corzide (nadolol 40 mg with a diuretic bendroflumethiazide 5 mg) might be used as initial therapy. Utilizing combination therapy should result in goal blood pressure in about 65% to 70% of subjects, whereas monotherapy might only be successful in about 40% to 50%.

24-hour BP load (**Figure 4.4**). Although ambulatory BP measurements might theoretically be useful in such patients, this is often impractical and may be unnecessary.

More practical are home BP measurements by the patient. If home BP measurements are to be meaningful, it is important that the care provider confirm both the validity of the instrument and the technique used by patients in making these measurements. BPs should be measured with a calibrated mercury or aneroid sphygmomanometer on three separate office visits to ascertain an appropriate baseline BP unless the first one or two BPs are ≥160/100 mm Hg, in which case a diagnosis of hypertension is justified. Most home BP aneroid or electronic monitors are accurate; finger monitors are probably less so and should be avoided. Because diabetics often are "nondippers" and the daytime BP may not reflect the pressure load imposed on the cardiovascular (CV) system and the kidneys (ie, an office BP of 140/90 mm Hg may be of greater significance in these patients than in a nondiabetic subjects whose BPs are lower at night). Elevations of nocturnal BPs, especially SBP, may disproportionately increase cardiovascular disease (CVD) risk as well as progression of renal disease in these patients. BPs should be measured in the standing position as well as the seated position because diabetics are more likely to have significant orthostatic decreases in their BP. The standing BP is important when titrating therapy. As noted in Chapter 1, *Introduction*, the Seventh Joint National Committee on Prevention, Detection, Evaluation, and Treatment of High Blood Pressure (JNC 7) has designated BP between 120/80 and 139/89 mm Hg as "prehypertensive." While these levels of BP may not require specific therapy in patients without CV risk factors, some therapy may be required in diabetics.

Essential hypertension is the major form of elevated BP in diabetic patients. Younger diabetics do not appear to have an increase in secondary forms of hypertension. Because diabetes is more common with increasing age, the physician should be aware of the possibility of renal artery atherosclerosis, a condition that also should be considered in other elderly patients, especially if the patient has been or is currently a smoker. Obviously, it is important to obtain a serum creatinine, electrolytes, and a spot urine albumin and creatinine for determination of the presence of microalbuminuria. It should be remembered that renal disease, which occurs in approximately 20% of patients with type 2 diabetes and in one third of those with type 1 diabetes, is an important predictor of progression of hypertension in these patients. The presence of microalbuminuria indicates that the patient is at greater risk for a myocardial infarction (MI) and stroke as well as the progression of renal disease. Therefore, the presence of microalbuminuria necessitates more rigorous control of BP and other CV risk factors as indicated in the guidelines from JNC 7 and from the American Diabetes Association (ADA). The presence of a creatinine level of >1.5 mg/dL is also an indication for more aggressive therapy. BP levels of 120/75 mm Hg would be an appropriate therapeutic target in such patients.

Therapy in patients with hypertension and diabetes should include lifestyle modifications involving weight reduction, increased aerobic activity, and moderation of salt and alcohol intake (**Table 7.1**). Most experts believe that medications should be started at the same time as lifestyle interventions in these patients since diabetics, even with stage or grade 1 hypertension, are in a high-risk category (**Table 7.2**). Most diabetics with definite elevations of BP will require medication to achieve goal BP. Based on previously described clinical trial results, angiotensin-converting enzyme (ACE) inhibitors, low-dose diuretics, β-blockers, calcium channel blockers (CCBs), and angiotensin II receptor blockers (ARBs) may be effective first-line

---

TABLE 7.1 — Lifestyle Modifications for Control of Hypertension and/or Overall Cardiovascular Risk

- Weight loss, if overweight*
- Reduction of sodium intake to <100 mmol/day (2.4 g sodium or approximately 6 g sodium chloride)*
- Limit alcohol intake to <1 oz/day of ethanol (24 oz beer, 10 oz wine, or 2 oz 80-proof whiskey); approximately one half of these amounts for women and thin people
- Cessation of smoking and reduction of dietary saturated fat and cholesterol for overall cardiovascular health; reduced fat intake also helps reduce caloric intake—important for control of weight and type 2 diabetes
- Maintain adequate dietary potassium, calcium, and magnesium intake
- Relaxation techniques—biofeedback
- Vegetarian diets, fish oil

* These interventions have been found to be most effective. Data on other interventions are not definitive (see text).

Modified from: The JNC 7 Report. *JAMA*. 2003;289:2560-2572.

TABLE 7.2 — Risk Stratification of Hypertension to Guide Treatment Choices*†

Blood Pressure Stages (mm Hg)	Initial Therapy‡		
	Risk Group A (No risk factors; no TOD/CVD)	**Risk Group B** (At least one risk factor, *not including diabetes*; no TOD/CVD)	**Risk Group C** (TOD or evidence of CVD and/or diabetes, with/without other risk factors)§
Prehypertension (120-139/80-89)	Lifestyle modification	Lifestyle modification	Possibly medication
Stage 1 (140-159/90-99)	Lifestyle modification (up to 4-6 months)	Lifestyle modification‖ (up to 2-3 months)	Medication plus lifestyle changes
Stage 2 (≥160/≥100)	Medication	Medication	Medication

Abbreviations: CVD, cardiovascular disease; JNC 7, Seventh Joint National Committee on the Prevention, Detection, Evaluation and Treatment of High Blood Pressure; LVH, left ventricular hypertrophy; TOD, target-organ disease.

* Modified from JNC-7
† *Lifestyle modification should be adjunctive therapy for all patients recommended for pharmacologic therapy.*
‡ For example, a patient with diabetes and a blood pressure of 142/94 mm Hg plus LVH should be classified as having stage 1 hypertension with TOD (LVH) and with another major risk factor (diabetes). Patient would be *Stage 1, Risk Group C*; pharmacologic treatment should be initiated at the same time as lifestyle modifications.
§ Any patient with diabetes should be considered in the same category as a patient with CVD and treated with medication in addition to lifestyle modifications.
‖ For patients with multiple risk factors, clinicians should consider drugs as initial therapy plus lifestyle modifications.

therapy in these patients. But most hypertensive diabetic patients will need more than one agent and most often a diuretic is needed to achieve the therapeutic BP goal of 130/85 mm Hg. For that reason, JNC 7 suggests the use of the two medications as appropriate initial therapy in diabetic hypertensives, especially patients with BP >160/100 mm Hg.

Nonpharmacologic Treatment

The first approach to the treatment of hypertension in diabetics, as well as in nondiabetics, should be lifestyle modifications. Estimates of how much BP might be lowered by lifestyle changes are listed in **Table 7.3**. In some cases, this degree of BP change will represent adequate treatment, but most patients with hypertension will require medication to achieve goal BP.

Initial efforts should include weight loss, if appropriate. Weight reduction is probably the single most important nondrug intervention. This may be especially

TABLE 7.3 — Lifestyle Modifications	
	Approximate SBP Reduction (Range/mm Hg)
Weight reduction	5-20/10 kg of weight loss
DASH eating plan	8-14
Dietary sodium reduction	2-8
Physical activity	4-9
Moderation of alcohol consumption	2-4
Abbreviations: DASH, Dietary Approaches to Stop Hypertension; SBP, systolic blood pressure.	
The JNC 7 Report. *JAMA*. 2003;289:2560-2572.	

important in diabetic subjects. Obesity is present in >60% of diabetics and hyperlipidemia is also a common finding. Losing weight and reducing lipid levels should be a major priority. But most people are unaware of their so-called ideal weight and when they are told to lose weight, they do not have a good idea of a goal or ideal weight. Of course, looking in a mirror will often help to determine whether or not someone is overweight, but there are more scientific and quite simple ways to do this.

Although body mass index (BMI) is used by many physicians to define overweight or obesity and target BMIs are set for patients, this is often confusing. **Table 7.4** outlines how to calculate the BMI and defines the limits of normal. A more simple method that is reasonably accurate in calculating ideal weight is noted in **Table 7.5**. These numbers are not set in granite and a variance of 5 to 10 lb is reasonable.

The next question is How many calories does a patient need to maintain weight or lose weight? Again, a simple formula is helpful (**Table 7.6**). With these guidelines, the patient and physician may embark on a reasonable diet program. Even a 10-lb weight loss may result in a decrease in BP so that specific medication may not be necessary. Weight loss will frequently help to reduce lipid levels and will increase insulin sensitivity and help to control blood glucose levels.

While maintaining an ideal weight or losing weight is an appropriate first step in all hypertensive individuals, it is especially important in diabetics. A low-calorie, low–saturated-fat diet should therefore be advised. Recent data also indicate that maintaining appropriate weight or losing weight may actually prevent the development of hypertension. Diabetic patients should consult their physicians before going on one of the recently popular low-carbohydrate or high-protein, high-fat diets. To reemphasize, people may lose

TABLE 7.4 — Calculating Body Mass Index and Desirable Ranges

Body mass index (BMI) = $\dfrac{\text{Weight in kilograms}}{\text{Height in meters squared}}$

To convert pounds to meters, divide by 2.2.

Example: $\dfrac{220 \text{ pound man}}{2.2} = 100$ kg

To convert height in inches to meters, divide by 39.4

Example: $\dfrac{74 \text{ inches}}{39.4} = 1.9$ meters [squared = 3.6]

To calculate the BMI of a man 1.9 meters tall and weighing 100 kg:

$\dfrac{100 \text{ kg}}{3.6} = \text{BMI} = 28$

	BMI	
	Men	**Women**
Desirable range	22-24	21-23
Overweight	>28	>27
Seriously overweight	>32-33	>31

weight while on these diets but there are very few data on their long-term effects. There are abundant data, for example, to suggest that people on a high-fat diet are at increased risk of heart disease. It should be remembered that most diabetic hypertensive individuals will require one or more antihypertensive drugs in addition to lifestyle changes to lower their BP to goal levels.

A decrease in sodium (salt) intake is also indicated despite recent controversies about the benefits of salt restriction. Data link a high salt intake to elevated BP and lower intake to some reduction in BP. Diabetics appear to be salt sensitive; BP responds to salt restriction to a greater degree in these individuals, especially

TABLE 7.5 — Simple Method of Calculating Ideal Weight*

Women
  100 lb for first 5 ft of height
  plus 5 lbs for each additional inch
  Example:
    5' 5" woman = 100 + (5 × 5) = 125 lb

Men
  106 lb for first 5 ft of height
  plus 6 lb for each additional inch
  Example:
    6' man = 106 + (12 × 6) = 178 lb

* Plus or minus 5 to 10 lb.

TABLE 7.6 — Calculating Calories to Maintain or Lose Weight

Calculating daily caloric intake necessary to maintain ideal body weight:

  Ideal weight × Level of physical activity

Example: maintaining ideal weight of 125 lb…

Sedentary 13	125 × 13 = 1625 cal/d
Moderately active 15	125 × 15 = 1875 cal/d
Active 17	125 × 17 = 2125 cal/d

Calculating daily caloric intake reduction necessary to lose weight:

Reducing caloric intake by 500 cal/d will result in weight loss of 1 lb/wk (500 × 7 = 3500 cal/wk), or reduce intake by 300 cal/d and exercise to burn off 200 cal/d.

Example: If a moderately active individual can maintain body weight with 1875 cal/d, a 500 cal/d reduction over 1 week will be necessary to lose 1 lb of body weight (1875 − 500 = 1375 cal/d × 7 days).

if they are >60 years of age, than in many other hypertensive subjects. Therefore, limitation of sodium intake is especially important in diabetics if they have hypertension (BP >140/90 mm Hg or even lower BP of 130-135/80-85 mm Hg). Restriction need not be severe; most patients will not tolerate a very low-sodium diet for long periods of time. A limited intake of heavily salted foods—pretzels, salted peanuts, hot dogs, processed meats, canned soups, etc—and limitation of salt in cooking and at the table will probably reduce intake to the presently recommended 6 g of salt (2.4 g sodium) per day. A good rule in selecting prepared foods is to avoid (if possible) foods with a sodium content of >150 mg per serving—*read labels*. **Table 7.7** lists foods to be avoided or markedly limited (see Chapter 10, *Cardiovascular Risk Reduction: Control of Diabetes*, for a review of lifestyle changes that should be made in all diabetics).

Recent data suggest that further limitations to 1.5 g of sodium per day will reduce BP to a greater degree. This level of restricted intake is more difficult

TABLE 7.7 — Some High–Sodium-Content Foods That Should Be Avoided

- Potato chips
- Pretzels
- Salted crackers
- Biscuits
- Pancakes
- Fast foods
- Olives
- Pickles
- Sauerkraut
- Soy sauce
- Catsup
- Bouillon
- Ham
- Sausages
- Frankfurters
- Smoked meats or fish
- Sardines
- Tomato juice (canned)
- Frozen lima beans
- Frozen peas
- Canned spinach
- Canned carrots
- Many kinds of cheese
- Commercially prepared soups or stews
- Pastries or cakes made from self-rising flour mixes

to achieve because of the amount of processed food that people consume, but it might be possible without a drastic modification of diet. The Dietary Approaches to Stop Hypertension (DASH) diet, which is a balanced diet consisting of fruits, vegetables, and low-fat dairy products along with a low sodium content, is a reasonable diet for hypertensive diabetics to follow.

The JNC 7 has suggested BP levels <140/90 mm Hg as a goal for nondiabetic individuals, but levels of <130/80-85 mm Hg for diabetic patients. Evidence that has become available indicates that lower levels may be more effective in diabetic hypertensives in reducing CV events. Increasing evidence from recent trials has also led to the recommendations of a committee of the National Kidney Foundation and the ADA that BP goals in the diabetic should be <130/80-85 mm Hg or *as low as possible consistent with treatment that does not cause annoying symptoms.*

Pharmacologic Therapy

Once the decision has been made to treat a hypertensive diabetic patient with medication, a choice of initial therapy must be made. Diabetic hypertensives fall into the high-risk category, and the JNC 7, as well as other national committees, have recommended that medication be started initially along with lifestyle changes in these patients. Medication should be started at the same time as weight loss, a low-sodium diet, and an exercise program (**Table 7.2**).

Some physicians still believe that a trial of nonpharmacologic interventions alone is justified for a period of time ranging from 1 to 3 months, depending on the level of BP, but we agree with the JNC 7 approach. In addition, as noted, many of these individuals will not respond to goal levels of BP with one medication. It is therefore recommended by the JNC 7 committee that multiple agents (alone or in combination) can represent initial therapy. Among the medications that have proven effective in reducing BP as well as morbidity/mortality in diabetic hypertensives are the ACE inhibitors, diuretics, β-blockers, and more recently, the ARBs. Data on the CCBs are less definitive except in the elderly. These medications will reduce BP and reduce the occurrence of stroke, but some studies suggest that they may not be as effective as an ACE inhibitor plus a diuretic in reducing CHD events, progression of renal disease in diabetics, and especially heart failure. In the Antihypertensive and Lipid-Lowering Treatment to Prevent Heart Attack Trial (ALLHAT), which included 14,000 diabetic patients, there was no difference in primary coronary heart disease (CHD) outcome (fatal and nonfatal MIs) among the three agents tested (eg, ACE inhibitor, dihydropyridine CCB, and diuretic). There were, however, fewer cases of heart failure with the diuretic compared with the CCB.

In this 5-year trial, 9.8% of the CCB-treated patients developed new-onset diabetes (NOD) compared with 11.6% in the diuretic group and 8.1% in the ACE inhibitor group. The difference between the ACE inhibitor and diuretic groups was significant—the ACE inhibitor/CCB difference was 1.8% and not significant (**Table 5.3**).

A recent study, the Valsartan Antihypertensive Long-term Use Evaluation (VALUE) trial that evaluated an ARB-treated and a CCB-treated group of high-risk subjects also reported fewer NOD cases in the ARB group than in the CCB group (13.1% compared with 16.4%; $P = 0.0001$).

These new trials indicate that CHD morbidity and mortality rates in hypertensive patients and hypertensive diabetics are not significantly different when a CCB is used as baseline therapy when compared with rates in patients treated with an ARB or ACE inhibitor. However, there are data from other smaller trials

(Fosinopril vs Amlodipine Cardiovascular Events Trial [FACET], Appropriate Blood Pressure Control in Diabetes Trial [ABCD], African American Study of Kidney Disease and Hypertension [AASK], etc) that cannot be discounted and indicate a benefit of renin-angiotensin-aldosterone system (RAAS) inhibitors compared with CCB therapy in diabetic patients, especially those with any degree of nephropathy.

A suggested treatment program for patients with hypertension and type 2 diabetes is presented in **Figure 7.1**.

■ Angiotensin-Converting Enzyme Inhibitors

ACE inhibitors have been recommended as initial antihypertensive therapy in diabetic persons with proteinuria. These medications are usually given with a diuretic to gain better BP control. They have been shown to protect against deterioration of renal disease (diabetic nephropathy) as well as progression of proteinuria. These effects of ACE inhibitors have been observed in normotensive as well as hypertensive patients with diabetes. As repeatedly emphasized, it is now recognized that proteinuria is a predictor of CVD as well as diabetic nephropathy.

It is not surprising therefore that ACE inhibitor therapy has resulted in reductions in MI and stroke. As previously noted, a cardioprotective effect of ACE inhibitors over and above that which may be provided by CCBs in diabetic patients was suggested by the results of the smaller ABCD and FACET studies. In addition, the Captopril Prevention Project (CAPPP) and the Heart Outcomes Prevention Evaluation (HOPE) trials also demonstrated a reduction of CV events in diabetics with the use of an ACE inhibitor. The results of the HOPE and CAPPP trials indicate that the use of ACE inhibitors when added to other medications not only reduces macrovascular and microvascular disease in diabetic hypertensive patients but also may prevent the development of type 2 diabetes in hypertensive patients. This finding might have been anticipated since these patients are often insulin-resistant and have a 2- to 3-fold greater propensity to develop type 2 diabetes than normotensive persons. ACE inhibitor–induced improvement of insulin resistance may be explained by improved blood flow to the skeletal muscle microcirculation as well as improved insulin action at the tissue level. **Table 7.8** lists information about the available ACE inhibitors.

■ Angiotensin Receptor Blockers

Recent clinical trial data support the role of ARBs in high-risk patients, such as those with diabetes and hypertension. This is based on a number of factors. First, inhibition of converting enzyme by ACE inhibitors may not be sustained over time, as these agents are competitive inhibitors whose blockade may be overridden by increased angiotensin I levels. This may result from increased renin production as a result of the loss of feedback inhibition. In an unblocked renin system, the generation of angiotensin II tends to suppress renin production. If angiotensin II is not generated as a result of ACE inhibition, this feedback loop is interrupted, more renin is generated, and more angiotensin I is produced; this may overwhelm ACE blockade with some production of angiotensin II. Further, there is increasing evidence that alternative pathways of conversion of angiotensin I to angiotensin II may restore circulating or tissue levels of angiotensin II despite ACE inhibition. Indeed, circulating angiotensin II levels may return toward pretreatment levels during long-term ACE inhibitor therapy.

Angiotensin II receptor blockers competitively block the AT_1 receptor subtype in peripheral tissues. The AT_1 receptor mediates the known CV and renal effects of angiotensin II. Studies in animal models of diabetic renal disease have shown that ARBs, like ACE

TABLE 7.8 — ACE Inhibitors Used for Treating Hypertension

Generic (Trade) Name	Usual Dosage Range Dose (mg)	Usual Dosage Range Frequency	Adverse Reactions	Physiologic Effects	Comments
Benazepril (Lotensin)	10-40	1 or 2/day	*Cough*, rash, loss of taste, palpitations, rarely angioedema	Blocks formation of angiotensin II, promoting vasodilation and decreased aldosterone; also increases bradykinin and vasodilator prostaglandins	Diuretic doses should be reduced before starting angiotensin-converting enzyme (ACE) inhibitor whenever possible to prevent excessive hypotension. Smaller doses in patients with serum creatinine >3.0 mg/dL. May cause hyperkalemia in patients with renal impairment or in those receiving potassium-sparing agents. Can cause renal failure in patients with bilateral renal artery stenosis
Captopril (Capoten)	25-100	2/day			
Enalapril (Vasotec)	2.5-40	1 or 2/day			
Fosinopril (Monopril)	10-40	1/day			
Lisinopril (Zestril, Prinivil)	10-40	1/day			
Moexipril (Univasc)	7.5-30	1/day			
Perindopril (Aceon)	4-8	1 or 2/day			
Quinapril (Accupril)	10-40	1/day			
Ramipril (Altace)	2.5-20	1/day			
Trandolapril (Mavik)	1-4	1/day			

inhibitors, reduce the progression of microalbuminuria and renal dysfunction. A recent study in patients with diabetic renal disease confirmed that valsartan and the ACE inhibitor captopril are equally effective in decreasing urinary protein excretion. The recently reported trials with losartan and irbesartan confirm the beneficial effects of these agents in patients with either microproteinuria or >300 mg/day of proteinuria as well as in patients with elevated creatinine levels.

Diabetic patients with cardiomyopathy may also benefit from using an ACE inhibitor and ARB together. In the Randomized Evaluation of Strategies for Left Ventricular Dysfunction (RESOLV) trial, the combination of the ARB candesartan and the ACE inhibitor enalapril was well tolerated, but the study was not powered to evaluate effects on long-term outcome comparing the ARB or ACE inhibitor alone. Additional studies are ongoing to evaluate the impact of combinations of ARB and ACE inhibitor therapy on renal disease and CVD as well as on mortality in diabetic patients with hypertension.

ARBs are listed in JNC 7 as one of the initial therapies for hypertension in diabetic patients, and based on recent data, the ADA has recommended these agents as a preferred first-step drug in these patients. The Reduction of Endpoints in NIDDM With an Angiotensin II Antagonist, Losartan (RENAAL), the Irbesartan Diabetic Nephropathy Trial (IDNT), and the Irbesartan Microalbuminuria in Type 2 Diabetes Mellitus in Hypertensive Patients (IRMA 2) trial results all indicated that a program based on ARB therapy compared with a program not including an ARB will reduce the progression of renal disease from less severe to more severe and will reduce the progression to end-stage renal disease in type 2 hypertensive diabetics with proteinuria. The ability of the ARBs to reduce albuminuria suggests that these blocking agents may also protect against CVD. Recent trials with these agents, such as the Losartan Intervention for Endpoint Reduction in Hypertension study (LIFE), provide us with indications about the use of these drugs in reducing CVD in diabetic patients. The ARBs can be used instead of ACE inhibitors in diabetic patients, in part because of their excellent side-effect profile. We await more definitive data that the use of an ARB-based treatment program provides comparable CVD risk reduction over time in this high-risk group of patients. **Table 7.9** lists available ARBs.

The VALUE study was designed to answer the question as to whether the use of a regimen based on an ARB (valsartan 80-160 mg/day) would result in a better outcome than a regimen based on a CCB (amlodipine 5-10 mg/day) in a high-risk group of 15,245 patients (46% had evidence of CHD). Hydrochlorothiazide was added to help achieve goal BP. At the end of >4 years, there was no difference between groups in overall cardiac end points but some difference in specific events, ie, MIs were significantly lower (25.8%) in the CCB group.

Sixty-four percent of the CCB group and 58% of the ARB subjects achieved SBP <140 mm Hg, and there was a difference in BP levels, especially at 1 month and 6 months (–4/–2 mm Hg and –2.1/–1.6 mm Hg) with the CCB. In the opinion of the investigators, this was consistent with the outcome and further evidence that BP lowering, especially in the early months, makes a difference. When groups of patients with an equivalent decrease in BP were compared, there were no differences in outcome between the CCB and the ARB groups. As noted, however, a definite finding in the VALUE trial was the occurrence of fewer cases of NOD in the ARB group compared with the CCB patients.

■ Diuretics

Thiazide diuretics in relatively low doses (equivalent to about 25 mg/day hydrochlorothiazide or about

TABLE 7.9 — Angiotensin II Receptor Blockers Used for Treating Hypertension

Generic (Trade) Name	Usual Dosage Range Dose (mg)	Usual Dosage Range Frequency	Adverse Reactions	Physiologic Effects	Comments
Candesartan (Atacand)	8-32	1/day	Occasional dizziness; generally well tolerated	Blocks action of angiotensin II; → vasodilation; ↓ aldosterone secretion	Diuretic doses should be reduced before starting angiotensin II receptor blocker whenever possible to prevent excessive hypotension. Reduce dose in patients with serum creatinine >3.0 mg/dL. Can cause renal failure in patients with bilateral renal artery stenosis
Eprosartan (Teveten)	400-800	1 or 2/day			
Irbesartan (Avapro)	150-300	1/day			
Losartan (Cozaar)	25-100	1 or 2/day			
Olmesartan (Benicar)	20-40	1/day			
Telmisartan (Micardis)	20-80	1/day			
Valsartan (Diovan)	80-320	1/day			

15 mg/day chlorthalidone) are effective and safe antihypertensive agents in type 2 diabetic patients. In the Systolic Hypertension in the Elderly Program (SHEP) study, adults with type 2 diabetes derived at least as much benefit in stroke and coronary heart disease reduction as those without diabetes. Diuretics in relatively low doses are not generally associated with metabolic abnormalities. The use of a diuretic or diuretic/β-blocker–based regimen in several large trials (ie, STOP-2, United Kingdom Prospective Diabetes Study [UKPDS]) reduced morbidity/mortality and lowered BP to a degree equal to other antihypertensive agents in hypertensive diabetic subjects. These agents are often a necessary part of the antihypertensive regimen in diabetic patients because these patients are often salt sensitive and have expanded plasma volumes. A majority of diabetic patients will not achieve goal BPs of <130-135/80-85 mm Hg without the use of a diuretic. Information about available thiazide diuretics is listed in **Table 7.10**. Concerns about possible adverse effects of these agents on glucose metabolism are addressed in Chapter 5.

■ β-Blockers

β-Blockers are useful agents in the treatment of hypertension in diabetic patients. For many years, physicians were advised not to use these medications in diabetics or to use them with care. Recent trials, however, have confirmed that β-blockers are safe and effective in diabetic patients. In the UKPDS, an atenolol-based treatment program reduced microvascular complications of diabetes by 37%, stroke by 44%, and death related to diabetes by 32%. The atenolol regimen was equally as effective as a captopril-based program in reducing microvascular and macrovascular complications of diabetes. The ability of β-blockers to suppress the renin-angiotensin system may, in part, account for this beneficial result. β-Blockers are es-

TABLE 7.10 — Some Commonly Used Diuretics for Treating Hypertension

Diuretic Generic (Trade) Name	Recommended Dosage Range Dose (mg)	Recommended Dosage Range Frequency	Duration of Action (hours)	Comments
Thiazide and Related Agents				
Chlorthalidone (Hygroton) (Thalitone)	12.5-25 / 15	1/d / 1/d	24-72 / 24-72	More effective than loop diuretics except in patients with serum creatinine >2.5 mg/dL—hydrochlorothiazide or chlorthalidone were used in most clinical trials
Hydrochlorothiazide (HydroDIURIL, Microzide)	12.5-50	1-2/d	12-18	
Indapamide (Losol)	1.25-5.0	1/d	18-24	A relatively low-sodium and high-potassium diet may help to augment blood pressure lowering and prevent hypokalemia
Methyclothiazide (Enduron)	2.5-5	1/d	>24	
Metolazone (Mykrox, Zaroxolyn)	0.5-5	1/d	18-24	

pecially indicated in diabetic patients with known coronary artery disease.

Generally, there are no major problems with β-blockers with regard to worsening hyperglycemic control in causing or masking hypoglycemia in most patients with type 2 diabetes. The use of carvedilol, a β-blocker with vasodilating properties, has less effect on glucose metabolism than a β-blocker without α-blocking properties. Carvedilol has antioxidant and antiproliferative properties, is an effective BP-lowering agent, and does not increase vascular resistance. Some reports suggest an increase in the risk of developing hyperglycemia with the use of either a β-blocker or diuretic, but this was not noted when all of the antihypertensive agents were compared in a review of data in treated patients (**Figure 7.2**). While hypertensive individuals are at greater risk for developing diabetes than nonhypertensives, there was no difference in risk associated with different medications. In a prospective study of >12,000 patients, however, after adjustments for age, gender, activity level, family history, adiposity, etc), a 28% increase in NOD was found in patients taking a β-blocker compared with those not on any medication. In this study, risk was not increased in patients on a diuretic, ACE inhibitor, or CCB. The authors stated that "concern about this risk of diabetes should not discourage physicians from prescribing thiazide diuretics to nondiabetic adults who have hypertension. The use of β-blockers appears to increase the risk of diabetes, but this adverse effect must be weighed against the proven benefits of β-blockers in reducing the risk of CV events."

A recent randomized double-blind study, Glycemic Effects in Diabetic Mellitus: Carvedilol-Metoprolol Comparison in Hypertensives (GEMINI), evaluated 1235 type 2 diabetics with a mean age of 61 years. A 5-month maintenance period compared the use of metoprolol (average dose 128 mg bid) with carvedilol

FIGURE 7.2 — Risk of Hyperglycemia With Use of Antihypertensive Drugs

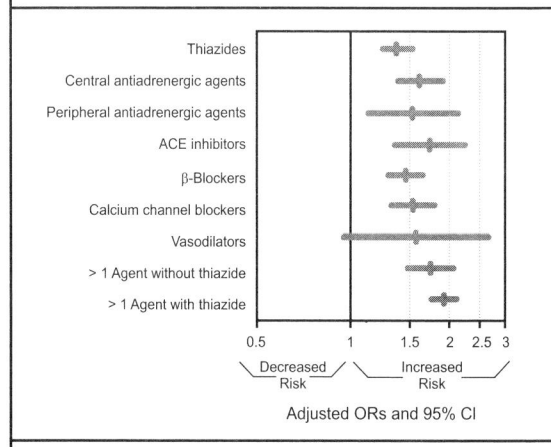

Abbreviations: ACE, angiotensin-converting enzyme; CI, cardiac index; OR, odds ratio.

Risk for development of hyperglycemia requiring treatment with antidiabetic drugs in users of antihypertensive drugs relative to nonusers. Note increased risk overall in hypertensive subjects compared with nonhypertensives, but no difference between drugs.

From: Gutwitz HJ, et al. *Ann Intern Med*. 1993;118:273-278.

(average dose 17.5 mg bid) when added to baseline therapy of an ACE inhibitor or an ARB (**Table 7.11**). Baseline BPs were 149/86 mm Hg and 149/87 mm Hg, respectively. More than 40% of patients required the addition of hydrochlorothiazide and >20% required a CCB to control BP. No BP or plasma glucose level differences were noted between the two groups. However, patients experienced statistically significantly more of an increase in HbA_{1c} with metoprolol (0.15%) than with carvedilol (0.02%)—a difference of 0.13%. Twice as many patients on metoprolol noted an increase in HbA_{1C} of 1.0%. The carvedilol group experienced an increase in insulin sensitivity, less progres-

TABLE 7.11 — GEMINI Study: Comparison of Carvedilol and Metoprolol in Diabetic Patients*

Study Outcome Measures	Carvedilol (n = 454) Baseline	Carvedilol (n = 454) 35 Weeks	Metoprolol (n = 657) Baseline	Metoprolol (n = 657) 35 Weeks	P Value = C/M
Mean BP (mm Hg)	149/87	131/77	149/86	132/77	NS
Plasma glucose (mg/dL)	147	155	147	157	NS
Mean Alb/Cr ratio	13	11	12	13	0.003
Triglycerides	159	168	168	186	<0.001
HbA$_{1c}$	**7.2**	**7.22**	**7.2**	**7.35**	**0.004**

Abbreviations: Alb, albumin; BP, blood pressure; Cr, creatinine; GEMINI, Glycemic Effects in Diabetes Mellitus: Carvedilol-Metoprolol Comparison in Hypertensives; HbA$_{1c}$, glycosylated hemoglobin; C/M, carvedilol compared with metoprolol.

* A study of 1235 patients aged 35-86 years with type 2 diabetes and hypertension who were also receiving an angiotensin-converting enzyme inhibitor (ACE-I) or an angiotensin II receptor blocker (ARB); >40% received hydrochlorothiazide and 25% received calcium channel blockers in order to achieve BP target.

Bakris GL, et al. *JAMA.* 2004;292:2227-2236.

sion to microalbuminuria, and significantly less of an increase in serum triglyceride levels.

This study confirms both the need for multiple medications to reduce BPs to goal levels in diabetic patients (even in those with less severe hypertension) and that a β-blocker with α-blocking capabilities may be preferred in diabetic patients because of its beneficial effect on glycemic control, insulin sensitivity, some of the manifestations of the metabolic syndrome, and the progression of albuminuria, which is frequently noted in type 2 diabetics and is a marker for systemic vascular disease.

Some concerns still exist, however, that β-blockers may cause hypoglycemia and mask symptoms of hypoglycemia in patients with type 1 diabetes and in type 2 diabetics with severe autonomic neuropathy. Available β-blockers and their dosing information are listed in **Table 7.12**.

■ Calcium Channel Blockers

Calcium channel blockers are often useful in conjunction with other drugs, particularly if diuretics, ACE inhibitors, or β-blockers alone or in combination are not effective in controlling the BP of a diabetic hypertensive. These agents were the initial therapeutic agents in the Systolic Hypertension in Europe Trial (Syst-Eur) and the Hypertension Optimal Treatment (HOT), both randomized trials. In both of these trials, diabetic persons had a significantly greater reduction in CVD events than did the nondiabetic hypertensive cohort. Most of these patients, as in all the other trials, required several medications to reach the more optimal SBP and diastolic blood pressure (DBP).

Some current recommendations suggest that CCBs are not the preferred medications for initial antihypertensive therapy, but should be considered as add-on or substitute therapy in those diabetics who cannot be controlled or cannot tolerate ACE inhibitors, β-block-

TABLE 7.12 — β-Blockers and Combined α_1/β-Blocker Used for Treating Hypertension*

Generic (Trade) Name	Usual Dosage Range* Dose (mg)	Frequency	Physiologic Effects	Comments
Atenolol[†] (Tenormin)	25-100	1/day	↓ cardiac output; ↓ plasma renin activity; ↓ blood pressure; ↓ pulse rate	Cardioselective agents may also inhibit β_2-receptors in higher doses (eg, all may aggravate asthma)
Bisoprolol[†] (Zebeta)	2.5-10	1/day		
Metoprolol[†] (Lopressor)	50-100	1 or 2/day		
Metoprolol XR[†] (Toprol-XL)	50-100	1/day		
Nadolol (Corgard)	40-120	1/day		
Propranolol LA (Inderal LA)	60-180	1/day		
Propranolol XL (InnoPran XL)	80-120	1/day (night)		
Timolol (Blocadren)	20-40	1/day		

β-Blockers With ISA[‡]			
Acebutolol[†] (Sectral)	200-800	2/day	Less effect on heart rate and vascular and bronchial smooth muscle	Possible advantage in subjects with bradycardia who require a β-blocker—they may produce fewer metabolic effects
Penbutolol (Levatol)	10-40	1/day		
Pindolol (Generic)	10-40	2/day		

Combined α₁ and β-Blocker			
Carvedilol (Coreg)	6.25-25	2/day	Cardiac output and renal blood flow maintained, blood pressure decreased. *antioxidant effects*	Beneficial effects in heart failure; may have less effect on glucose metabolism than other β-blockers

Abbreviations: LA, long acting; XR, extended release.

* Dosages may also differ from the manufacturer's prescribing information recommendations. These dosages are based on our experience and the belief that if small or moderate doses of one drug prove ineffective, small doses of a medication from another class should be added.

† Cardioselective.

‡ ISA = intrinsic sympathomimetic action (slight β_2-receptor stimulation).

ers, and/or diuretics. These agents are generally metabolically neutral. As noted, the VALUE and ALLHAT studies suggest that a long-acting dihydropyridine CCB is as effective as other agents in reducing BP and overall CHD events. As also noted, those medications may not be as effective in diabetic nephropathy or in preventing CHF. Short-acting dihydropyridine CCBs should not be used in diabetic patients because of the potential of increased CVD events in this high-risk population.

■ Combination Therapy and Combination Agents

In the large clinical trials that have demonstrated that diabetic patients benefit from rigorous lowering of SBP and DBP, at least two or three agents were necessary for optimal BP control. For example, in the UKPDS, approximately two thirds of the type 2 diabetic patients required multiple medications to achieve tight BP control of 144/82 mm Hg. In patients assigned to less-tight control (154/87 mm Hg), there was less frequent use of multiple antihypertensive agents and less reduction of macrovascular and microvascular risk. The results indicate that combination therapy with an ACE inhibitor or a β-blocker plus a diuretic may be more effective than monotherapy in reducing macrovascular and microvascular events, providing that BP is adequately lowered.

When ACE inhibitors are used in conjunction with low-dose diuretics, metabolic problems such as hyperkalemia (with ACE inhibitor alone) and hypokalemia/hypomagnesemia (with diuretics) are rare. β-Blockers and low-dose diuretics also represent good combination therapy in diabetic patients. The FACET trial provided some support for the use of an ACE inhibitor and CCB as combination therapy. The incidence of CVD was less in the group treated with the ACE inhibitor fosinopril than in the group that received the

CCB amlodipine, but the incidence of CVD events was least in the group that received both antihypertensive agents (**Figure 7.3**). The results suggest that ACE inhibitor and CCB combinations may be effective in reducing CVD risk in this population of diabetics with evidence of renal disease.

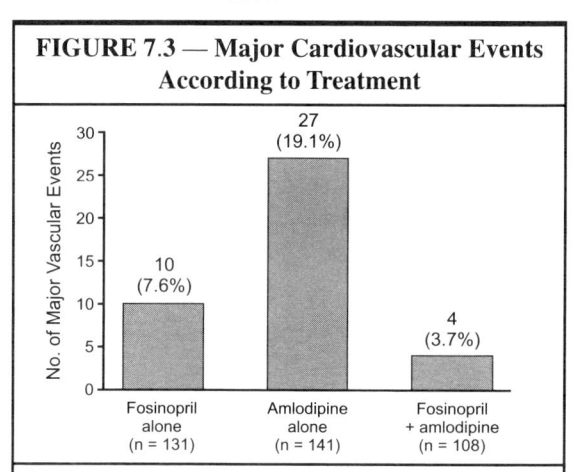

FIGURE 7.3 — Major Cardiovascular Events According to Treatment

Treatment	No. of Major Vascular Events
Fosinopril alone (n = 131)	10 (7.6%)
Amlodipine alone (n = 141)	27 (19.1%)
Fosinopril + amlodipine (n = 108)	4 (3.7%)

Cardiovascular events were reduced more with an angiotensin-converting enzyme (ACE) inhibitor than with a calcium channel blocker in the Fosinopril vs Amlodipine Cardiovascular Event Trial (FACET) in diabetics with evidence of renal disease. Best results were obtained when both agents were given together (small numbers of events).

Tatti P, et al. *Diabetes Care*. 1998;21:597-603.

In summary, once baseline ACE inhibitor therapy has been initiated and if goal BP has not been achieved, then combinations with low-dose diuretics, β-blockers, or CCBs represent an appropriate therapeutic approach to accomplish the BP goal of 130/80-85 mm Hg, and thus reduce macrovascular and microvascular disease in this high-risk population. Available combination hypertensive medications are listed in **Table 7.13**. In many cases, physicians may elect to

TABLE 7.13 — Combination Antihypertensive Medications

Generic Name	Trade Name	Available Dosages (mg)
ACE Inhibitors and Diuretics		
Benazepril/hydrochlorothiazide	Lotensin HCT	5/6.25, 10/12.5, 20/12.5, 20/25
Captopril/hydrochlorothiazide	Captozide*	25/15, 25/25, 50/15, 50/25
Enalapril/hydrochlorothiazide	Vaseretic	5/12.5, 10/25
Fosinopril/hydrochlorothiazide	Monopril HCT	10/12.5, 20/12.5
Lisinopril/hydrochlorothiazide	Prinzide; Zestoretic	10/12.5, 20/12.5, 20/25
Moexipril/hydrochlorothiazide	Uniretic	7.5/12.5, 15/12.5, 15/25
Quinapril/hydrochlorothiaizde	Accuretic	10/12.5, 20/12.5, 20/25
Angiotensin II Receptor Blockers and Diuretics		
Candesartan/hydrochlorothiazide	Atacand HCT	16/12.5, 32/12.5
Eprosartan/hydrochlorothiazide	Teveten HCT	600/12.5, 600/25
Irbesartan/hydrochlorothiazide	Avalide	150/12.5, 300/12.5
Losartan/hydrochlorothiazide	Hyzaar[†]	50/12.5, 100/25

Olmesartan/hydrochlorothiazide	Benicar HCT	20/12.5, 40/12.5, 40/25
Telmisartan/hydrochlorothiazide	Micardis HCT	40/12.5, 80/12.5
Valsartan/hydrochlorothiazide	Diovan HCT	80/12.5, 160/12.5, 160/25
β-Adrenergic Blockers and Diuretics		
Atenolol/chlorthalidone	Tenoretic	50/25, 100/25
Bisoprolol/hydrochlorothiazide	Ziac*	2.5/6.25, 5/6.25, 10/6.25
Metoprolol/hydrochlorothiazide	Lopressor HCT	50/25, 100/25, 100/50
Nadolol/bendroflumethiazide	Corzide	40/5, 80/5
Propranolol (XR)/hydrochlorothiazide	Inderide LA	80/50
Timolol/hydrochlorothiazide	Timolide	10/25
Calcium Channel Blockers and ACE Inhibitors		
Amlodipine/benazepril	Lotrel	2.5/10, 5/10, 5/20, 10/20
Felodipine/enalapril	Lexxel	2.5/5, 5/5
Trandolapril/verapamil XR	Tarka	2/180, 1/240, 2/240, 4/240

Continued

Generic Name	Trade Name	Available Dosages (mg)
Other Combinations		
Amiloride/hydrochlorothiazide	Moduretic	5/50
Clonidine/chlorthalidone	Clorpres	0.1/15, 0.2/15, 0.3/15
Methyldopa/hydrochlorothiazide	Aldoril	250/15, 250/25, 500/30, 500/50
Prazosin/polythiazide	Minizide	1/0.5, 2/0.5, 5/0.5
Reserpine/chlorthalidone	Diupres	250/0.125, 500/0.125
Reserpine/thiaizde	Hydropres	25/0.125, 50/0.125
Spironolactone/hydrochlorothiazide	Aldactazide	25/25, 50/50
Triamterene/hydrochlorothiazide	Dyazide, Maxzide	37.5/25, 75/50

Abbreviations: ACE, angiotensin-converting enzyme; XR, extended release

* Approved for initial therapy.
† Approved for initial therapy of severe hypertension (diastolic blood pressure ≥110 mm Hg).

start therapy in a diabetic hypertensive with a combination of an ACE inhibitor or an ARB plus a diuretic. This is the present recommendation of the JNC 7, especially if stage 2 hypertension is present (BP >160/100 mm Hg).

Specific Treatment Plan and Case Presentation

The treatment algorithm (**Figure 7.1**) can be used as a guide to management of the following case of diabetes and hypertension.

Case:

A 51-year-old woman with adult-onset (type 2) diabetes of 8 years' duration presents to a clinic for evaluation and optimization of therapy. Her diabetes was initially controlled on a sulfonylurea drug, but 2 years ago, metformin was added for better blood glucose control. She is overweight at 5'4" and 170 lb (ideal weight would be about 120-130 lb). She has been trying to lose weight, but has gained 2 lb over the past year. Her most recent fasting blood glucose levels are in the range of 110 to 140 mg/dL. Her BP was noted to be elevated 2 years prior to this visit and she has been taking amlodipine 5 mg/day with reported good BP control. She does not remember having her urine checked, having an electrocardiogram (ECG), or an eye exam. She has a family history of heart disease, kidney disease, and type 2 diabetes. She has gone through menopause over the past year and a half with hot flashes and a discontinuation of menstrual bleeding 6 to 9 months ago. She does not smoke and drinks moderately–one glass of wine every other day.

On physical examination, she is a pleasant, talkative, obese woman with some increase in central distribution of fat. Vital signs include a heart rate of 86 beats per minute and BP of 166/94 mm Hg. Funduscopic exam reveals grade 2 hypertensive changes (A-V nicking) with no evidence of proliferative diabetic retinopathy. There are no carotid bruits and the thyroid is of normal size. Cardiac exam reveals a normal rate and rhythm with an S_4 gallop at the apex, which is 2 cm lateral to the midclavicular line. Examination of the abdomen reveals no bruits or other abnormalities. Peripheral pulses are normal and no abnormal neurologic findings are evident.

Initial testing includes an ECG that is normal except for voltage criteria of left ventricular hypertrophy (LVH) and a spot urine albumin to creatinine level of 3.5 mg/mmol (normal, <2.0). Fasting glucose is 118 mg/dL and a fasting lipid profile reveals total cholesterol of 243 mg/dL, high-density lipoprotein (HDL) 32 mg/dL, triglycerides 220 mg/dL, and low-density lipoprotein (LDL) cholesterol 162 mg/dL. Serum creatinine is 1.1 mg/dL, and electrolytes are normal. Goals for this woman's management should include the following:

- In conjunction with a dietitian, a diet should be planned, and increased walking as a suitable form of aerobic exercise encouraged. Since she does not have a history of angina, an exercise ECG test or an exercise thallium scan is not indicated unless she plans to embark on a much more vigorous exercise program.
- If she can tolerate aspirin, she should be placed on a minimal dose 81 mg of aspirin daily.
- Since diet and exercise will lower her LDL by only about 25% at a maximum, or to levels of about 120-130 mg/dL, she should be placed on a 3-hydroxy-3-methylglutaryl coenzyme A (HMG-CoA) reductase inhibitor with the goal of lowering her LDL to <100 mg/dL.
- Given her inadequate BP control, LVH, and albuminuria, she should be placed on an ACE inhibitor or an ARB, which should be titrated at

least once if no side effects occur. As she has previously been taking amlodipine, it would be appropriate to continue that along with the ACE inhibitor. Given her relatively high SBP, a third agent (low-dose diuretic) will probably be needed to lower the SBP to ≤130 mm Hg and to reduce albuminuria. It would be appropriate to check the creatinine and potassium 2 to 4 weeks after initiating ACE inhibitor therapy. A slight rise in creatinine at 2 to 4 weeks might occur, but unless there is severe volume depletion or in the rare case where the patient has renal artery stenosis, the creatinine level should not rise significantly and should return to baseline or below the initial level over time. The increase in ACE inhibitor dosages and the addition of other agents may be accomplished over 1 to 2 months. It would be useful for the physician and educational for this patient if she would purchase a home BP measurement device and have it and her technique for measuring BP validated by the physician. This usually is motivational to the patient, as is home glucose monitoring, and provides additional data to the physician to assist him/her in adjusting the BP regimen over time.

This multifaceted approach to therapy is of great importance in reducing CV events and renal disease progression. *Glycemic control alone is not enough.*

SELECTED READING

Bakris GL, Williams M, Dworkin L, et al for the National Kidney Foundation Hypertension and Diabetes Executive Committees Working Group. Preserving renal function in adults with hypertension and diabetes: a consensus approach. *Am J Kidney Dis.* 2000;36:646-661.

Bakris GL, Fonseca V, Katholi RE, et al; GEMINI Investigators. Metabolic effects of carvedilol vs metoprolol in patients with type 2 diabetes mellitus and hypertension: a randomized controlled trial. *JAMA.* 2004;292:2227-2236.

Gress TW, Nieto FJ, Shahar E, Wofford MR, Brancati FL. Hypertension and antihypertensive therapy as risk factors for type 2 diabetes mellitus. Atherosclerosis Risk in Communities Study. *N Engl J Med.* 2000;342:905-912.

Grundy SM, Benjamin IJ, Burke GL, et al. Diabetes and cardiovascular disease: a statement for healthcare professionals from the American Heart Association. *Circulation.* 1999;100:1134-1146.

Lindholm LH, Ibsen H, Dahlof B, et al for the LIFE Study Group. Cardiovascular morbidity and mortality in patients with diabetes in the Losartan Intervention for Endpoint Reduction in Hypertension study (LIFE): a randomised trial against atenolol. *Lancet.* 2002;359:1004-1010.

Moser M. *Clinical Management of Hypertension.* 7th ed. Caddo, Okla: Professional Communications, Inc; 2004.

Moser M. Drug treatment of hypertension in the elderly and in diabetics. In: Van Zwieten PA, Greenlee WJ, eds. *Antihypertensive Drugs.* The Netherlands: Haswood Academic Publishers; 1997.

Moser M. Treating hypertension: calcium channel blockers, diuretics, beta-blockers, ACE inhibitors. Is there a difference? *J Clin Hypertens.* 2000;2:301-304.

Sowers JR. Treatment of hypertension in patients with diabetes. *Arch Intern Med.* 2004;164:1850-1857.

Sowers JR, Reed J. 1999 clinical advisory treatment of hypertension and diabetes. *J Clin Hypertens.* 2000;2:132-133.

The Seventh Report of the Joint National Committee on prevention, detection, evaluation, and treatment of high blood pressure. *JAMA.* 2003;289:2560-2572.

8 Cardiovascular Risk Reduction: Lipid-Lowering Therapy

Diabetic subjects without a prior myocardial infarction (MI) have almost the same risk of death as nondiabetic individuals who previously have had an MI; an aggressive approach to the management of all known risk factors is warranted. Dyslipidemia should be one of the targets to correct. The nature of the metabolic defects in lipid and lipoprotein metabolism differs between types 1 and 2 diabetes. The most typical lipoprotein pattern observed in type 2 diabetes consists of:

- Decreased high-density lipoprotein (HDL) levels (<45 mg/dL)
- High-normal or slightly elevated low-density lipoprotein (LDL) levels
- Hypertriglyceridemia, usually due to elevated triglyceride-rich, very low-density lipoprotein (VLDL) levels
- Increased small, dense LDL particles and increased intermediate-density lipoprotein (IDL) particles, both of which contribute disproportionately to atherogenic risk
- Total cholesterol is usually normal to slightly elevated.

A similar lipoprotein pattern can be seen in type 1 diabetic patients with nephropathy and in some patients after weight gain in association with intensive insulin treatment. Treated type 1 diabetic patients often have normal lipids and lipoproteins, although hypertriglyceridemia may be the result of inadequate glycemic control.

The main cause of hypertriglyceridemia in treated type 2 diabetic patients is an overproduction of VLDL. Low HDL cholesterol levels are partly due to a replacement of cholesterol in the core of HDL by triglycerides when hypertriglyceridemia is present. HDL levels also may be decreased as a result of impaired catabolism of VLDL. Both LDL and HDL particles are altered by hepatic lipase that is essential for triglyceride catabolism and for normal HDL production. Reduced activity of lipoprotein lipase is an important cause of hypertriglyceridemia in untreated patients. Complications such as nephropathy and the nephrotic syndrome can alter plasma lipid and lipoprotein levels with resultant elevations of total cholesterol.

Because of the atherogenic lipid profile of diabetic patients and their higher risk for cardiovascular disease (CVD), all type 2 diabetic patients should be screened for lipid abnormalities at the initial evaluation using a fasting lipid profile to determine serum total cholesterol, triglycerides, and HDL cholesterol. LDL cholesterol is then calculated from the formula: LDL = total cholesterol – HDL – (triglycerides divided by 5) if triglycerides are <400 mg/dL (otherwise the formula is inaccurate).

All adult type 2 diabetic patients should have their LDL cholesterol lowered to <100 mg/dL, their HDL raised >45 mg/dL, and triglycerides lowered to <150 mg/dL, if at all possible. This goal is similar to the secondary prevention goal in patients with known CVD.

Abnormal lipid levels have been identified as having a major impact on events related to atherosclerosis; levels that may be of limited significance in a nondiabetic may be of great significance in a diabetic. The Insulin Resistance Atherosclerosis Study (IRAS), which included patients with type 2 diabetes with both impaired and normal glucose tolerance, confirmed that dyslipidemia is a major risk factor for atherosclerosis. Although associations were found between lipoprotein concentrations and internal and common carotid artery thickness, these associations did not substantially differ among persons with and without diabetes. However, while the event rate in the nondiabetic is about 10 to 15 cardiovascular (CV) events per 10,000 person-years with a cholesterol level of about 210 mg/dL, a total cholesterol level of the same magnitude would translate into about 75 events per 10,000 person-years in a diabetic.

Approach to Prevention and Management of Atherosclerosis in Diabetes

The treatment of dyslipidemia in diabetes consists in part of improvement in diabetic control with diet, exercise, and pharmacologic therapy. The National Cholesterol Education Program (NCEP) has published a dietary recommendation that involves the restriction of dietary fat and cholesterol (**Table 8.1**). This diet, which also utilizes salt restriction, could be considered to be a relatively heart-smart diet for diabetics.

In view of the important role of lipids and lipoproteins in CVD and their frequent derangement in diabetes, it is not surprising that aggressive lipid management of the diabetic patient has been associated with a reduction in clinical events in patients with preexisting CVD. A major benefit appears to result from the use of 3-hydroxy-3-methylglutaryl coenzyme A (HMG-CoA) reductase inhibitors or statins, despite the fact that LDL levels, the lipid fraction primarily affected by these agents, are not usually increased in diabetics. Subgroup analysis of recent clinical trials in which statins have been used indicate that the reduction in events with statins is at least as great in dia-

TABLE 8.1 — Diet Recommendations for the Treatment of Lipid Disorders in Diabetes

- Calorie restriction for weight loss as indicated
- Total fat intake <30% of kcal, mostly monounsaturated (eg, canola oil, olive oil)*
- Saturated fat intake <7% of total kcal
- Total cholesterol intake <200 mg/day
- Carbohydrate intake 50% to 60% of total calories, emphasizing complex carbohydrates (at least five portions per day of fruits/vegetables); soluble fibers (legumes, oats, certain fruits/vegetables) have additional benefits on total cholesterol, low-density lipoprotein (LDL) cholesterol level, and glycemic control
- Sodium restriction ≤2400 mg/day for type 2 diabetic patients with hypertension; sodium restriction <2000 mg/day for type 2 diabetic patients with hypertension and nephropathy

* A reduction of total fat to below 20% to 25% of total calories is achievable and probably a better target than 30% of total calories on a 2000-cal/d diet. This suggests an intake of 400 to 500 calories as fat or between 45 and 55 g/fat/d (eg, 45 × 9 cal/g of fat = 405 cal). Food labels will help to guide this level of intake.

betic as in nondiabetic subjects. Lowering blood pressure (BP) (if elevated), reducing lipid levels (if elevated), and correcting coagulation abnormalities have been shown to improve CVD outcomes in diabetic patients. The clinical trials that have demonstrated significant CVD risk reduction with control of BP are addressed in Chapter 6, *Results of Hypertension Treatment Trials in Diabetic Patients*. Treatment of lipid abnormalities and platelet and coagulation treatment strategies are reviewed here.

In three secondary prevention studies using HMG-CoA reductase inhibitors (statins), a significant reduction in coronary and stroke events was noted in diabetic patients. In the Heart Protection Study (HPS),

5963 adults with diabetes were randomized to receive simvastatin 40 mg daily or matching placebo. There was a significant 22% reduction in the event rate in the simvastatin group for:
- Major coronary events
- Strokes
- Revascularizations.

Specifically, simvastatin treatment decreased coronary mortality by 20% and first nonfatal MI by 37%. There was a 24% reduction in nonfatal and fatal strokes. Allocation to the statin produced a 19% reduction in peripheral macrovascular complications, defined as any peripheral artery surgery, angioplasty, leg amputation, or leg ulcer. These positive results of cholesterol-lowering therapies were in addition to other treatments (ie, ACE inhibitors, β-blockers, and aspirin). The benefits extended to subjects with relatively normal LDL levels <116 mg/dL to both men and women and diabetic patients >65 years of age at entry.

In the Anglo-Scandinavian Cardiac Outcomes Trial (ASCOT), the reduction in stroke in diabetic subjects was 27% in 2,532 hypertensive patients with diabetes without previous CVD. In a recent landmark study of type 2 diabetic patients without elevated LDL cholesterol or prior CVD, the Collaborative Atorvastatin Diabetes Study (CARDS), patients randomized to atorvastatin 10 mg had a 36% reduction in acute coronary events and a striking 48% reduction in stroke compared with patients who were not treated with atorvastatin. These observations indicate that most patients with diabetes should receive statins, even if their LDL cholesterol is <100 mg/dL.

Some studies have been performed using fibrates, such as gemfibrozil (Lopid) or fenofibrate (Tricor), which theoretically may be more ideally suited to use in diabetic dyslipidemia. These studies have indicated that fibrates have a beneficial effect in diabetic subjects.

Niacin is the most effective drug for raising HDL, but in high doses may raise blood glucose and cause disturbing side effects (eg, headaches and flushing). Smaller doses (750-2000 mg/day), however, have been shown to have beneficial effects on LDL, HDL, and triglycerides with only small changes in blood glucose. These are generally amenable to adjustment of diabetic therapy. Combination therapy, with a statin and a fibrate, statin, or niacin, may be efficacious for patients needing treatment for all three lipid functions.

Generally, pharmacologic therapy is instituted along with diet therapy for the aggressive lowering of lipids in patients with diabetes. A mainstay of therapy is an HMG-CoA reductase inhibitor (ie, atorvastatin, fluvastatin, lovastatin, pravastatin, rosuvastatin, and simvastatin). These drugs inhibit cholesterol synthesis, up-regulate LDL receptors, and may help stabilize vulnerable atherosclerotic plaques, which are more prevalent and lethal in patients with diabetes. If additional triglyceride lowering is indicated, a fibric acid derivative such as gemfibrozil or fenofibrate can be added.

As both statins and fibrates have been shown to reduce the risk of CV events, the use of combination therapy may achieve additional risk reduction over and above that achieved with statin monotherapy. Because the combination is more likely to cause liver function abnormalities as well as myopathies, the creatine phosphokinase (CPK) and liver function should be monitored more closely. Once a stable and effective dose of the combination is reached and CPK and liver function tests are less than three times the upper limit of normal, then monitoring becomes less necessary. Dosing information on these lipid-lowering drugs is presented in **Table 8.2**.

Clinical Trials of Lipid Lowering in Diabetic Subjects

No clinical trial has been done on the effects of lipid-lowering agents on subsequent coronary heart disease (CHD) events specifically in diabetic subjects. A number of clinical trials have included adult type 2 diabetic subjects. In the Scandinavian Simvastatin Survival Study (4S) trial, simvastatin (Zocor) (HMG-CoA reductase inhibitor or statin) significantly reduced CHD incidence and total mortality (borderline significance) in diabetic subjects with high LDL cholesterol and with previous clinical CHD (**Figure 8.1**). In the Cholesterol and Recurrent Events (CARE) study, pravastatin (Pravachol) reduced CHD incidence significantly in diabetic subjects with average LDL levels and with previous clinical CHD. In the Long-Term Intervention With Pravastatin in Ischaemic Disease (LIPID) trial, pravastatin treatment reduced mortality and nonfatal MI in diabetic subjects with prior MI or hospitalization for unstable angina to a somewhat lesser degree than in nondiabetic subjects. In the Helsinki Heart Study, gemfibrozil (fibric acid derivative) was associated with a nonstatistically significant reduction in CHD in diabetic subjects without prior CHD. In the Veterans Affairs High-Density Lipoprotein Cholesterol Intervention Trial (VA-HIT), gemfibrozil was associated with a 24% decrease in CV events in diabetic subjects with CVD. **Table 8.3** summarizes the results of various intervention studies to lower lipids in patients with diabetes. The number necessary to treat (NNT) to prevent one CV event is listed in the last column.

Both 4S and CARE showed substantial benefits of statin therapy in the diabetic population with evidence of CHD. The results indicate that the effect of LDL cholesterol lowering on the risk of death, major CHD events, and any atherosclerotic event is similar

TABLE 8.2 — Lipid-Lowering Drugs: Preparations and Usual Dosing Regimens

Drug (Trade Name)	Availability	Starting Dose	Dose Range
Cholestyramine (Questran, Questran Light, Prevalite)	Powder for oral suspension: single-dose (4 g) packets or cans with dosing scoop (1 scoop = 1 dose)	4 g/d (1 scoop)	4-12 g bid
Colestipol (Colestid)	Granules: single-dose (5 g) packets or bottles with dosing scoop (1 scoop = 1 dose) Tablet: 1 g	5 g/d (1 scoop)	5-15 g bid
Colesevelam (WelChol)	Tablet: 625 mg	6 tablets/d	7 tablets/d (qd or bid)
Ezetimibe (Zetia)	Tablet: 10 mg	10 mg/d	10 mg/d
Gemfibrozil (Lopid)	Tablet: 600 mg	600 mg bid	600 mg bid
Fenofibrate (Tricor)	Tablet: 54, 160 mg	48-145 mg/d	48-145 mg/d
Nicotinic acid			
Immediate-release (Niacor, others)	Tablet: 5, 100, 250, 500, 1000 mg	50 mg tid	500-2000 mg tid

Sustained-release (Niaspan, Slo-Niacin, others)	Tablet: 250, 375, 500, 750, 1000 mg	500 mg/d	1000-2000 mg/d
Fish oil	Capsule: 1 g	3 g tid	2-6 g tid
HMG-CoA Reductase Inhibitors			
Atorvastatin (Lipitor)	Tablet: 10, 20, 40, 80 mg	10 mg/d	10-80 mg/d
Fluvastatin (Lescol) (Lescol XL)	Capsule: 20, 40 mg Tablet, ER: 80	20-40 mg qpm	20-40 mg qpm, 40 mg bid; for ER tablet, 80 mg qpm
Lovastatin (Altocor) (Mevacor)	Tablet, ER: 10, 20, 40, 60 mg Tablet: 10, 20, 40 mg	20 mg qpm 20 mg qpm	10-40 mg qpm, 40 mg bid
Pravastatin (Pravachol)	Tablet: 10, 20, 40, 80 mg	40 mg qpm	10-80 mg qpm
Rosuvastatin (Crestor)	Tablet: 5, 10, 20, 40 mg	5-20 mg/d	5-40 mg/d
Simvastatin (Zocor)	Tablet: 5, 10, 20, 40, 80 mg	20 mg qpm	5-80 mg qpm

Continued

Drug (Trade Name)	Availability	Starting Dose	Dose Range
Combinations			
Niacin/Lovastatin (Advicor)	Tablet: 500/20, 750/20, 1000/20 mg	500/20 qhs	500/20-2000/40 mg qhs
Ezetimibe/Simvastatin (Vytorin)	Tablet: 10/10, 10/20, 10/40, 10/80 mg	10/20 mg/d	10/10-10/80 mg/d
Abbreviation: ER, extended release; HMG-CoA, 3-hydroxy-3-methylglutaryl coenzyme A.			

FIGURE 8.1 — Simvastatin vs Placebo: Curves for Probability of Remaining Free of a Major Coronary Heart Disease Event

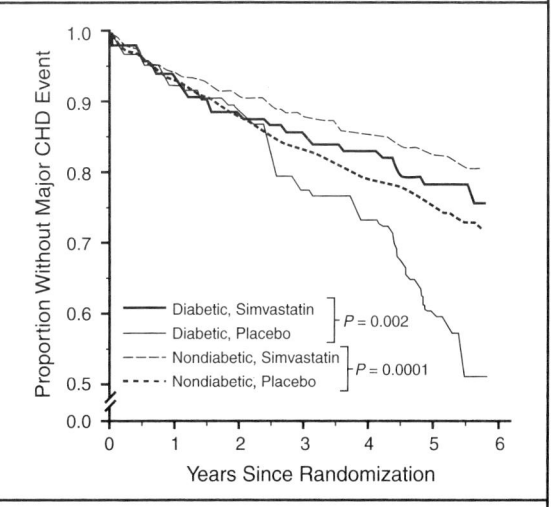

Survival curves for the probability of remaining free of a major coronary heart disease (CHD) event during follow-up in nondiabetic and diabetic patients treated with placebo or simvastatin. The Scandinavian Simvastatin Survival Study (4S) of patients with CHD. Note greater chance of survival without CHD event in both diabetics and nondiabetics in treated groups.

Pyörälä K, et al. *Diabetes Care*. 1997;20:614-620.

in diabetic and nondiabetic patients with CHD. Only 202 patients with diabetes were included in the 4S study. Simvastatin reduced major coronary events by 55% in the diabetic group and brought about reductions in total cholesterol of 27%; in LDL cholesterol, by 36%; and triglycerides by 11%; HDL cholesterol was increased by 7%.

The CARE trial included 586 patients with diabetes and demonstrated that pravastatin substantially reduced the incidence of a coronary event by 25% in

TABLE 8.3 — Reduction in Nonfatal MI or CAD Death in Patients With Diabetes Mellitus and CAD in Clinical Trials

Trial	n	CAD Events Placebo (%)	CAD Events Drug (%)	RR (%)	Absolute RR (%)	NNT to Prevent 1 Event
4S*	483	37.5	23.5	42	14.0	7
CARE/LIPID[†]	1368	22.1	18.6	17	3.5	29
VA-HIT[‡]	769	29.4	21.2	31	8.2	12

Abbreviations: CAD, coronary artery disease; CARE/LIPID, Cholesterol and Current Events [trial]/Long-term Intervention with Pravastatin in Ischemic Disease; NNT, number needed to treat; RR, relative risk; VA-HIT, Veterans Affairs High-Density Lipoprotein Intervention Trial.

* Includes patients with a history of diabetes or with fasting blood glucose ≥126 mg/dL at baseline.
† Combined CARE and LIPID trial results, published as the Pravastatin Pooling Project.
‡ Includes patients with a history of diabetes or with fasting blood glucose ≥126 mg/dL at baseline.

Adapted from: Robins SJ. *Am J Cardiol*. 2001;88(suppl):19N-23N.

patients with diabetes compared with 23% in those without diabetes (**Figure 8.2**). Because the risk of recurrent events is greater in diabetic than in nondiabetic patients with CHD, the absolute clinical benefit achieved by LDL cholesterol lowering may be greater in diabetic patients with CHD. The LIPID trial included 782 diabetics. Among the diabetic subgroup, death due to CHD and nonfatal MI were significantly reduced by 19% compared with 25% for nondiabetics. In the Air Force/Texas Coronary Atherosclerosis Prevention Study (AFCAPS/TexCAPS) primary prevention trial with lovastatin, the reduction of CVD events was significantly greater in the diabetic cohort.

Results of a study conducted in Italy suggest that treatment with an HMG-CoA reductase inhibitor may be useful for both primary and secondary prevention of chronic complications in patients with type 2 diabetes. In study subjects grouped according to CV risk, lipid profiles improved significantly during treatment with atorvastatin (Lipitor), generally in doses of 10 mg/day. In addition, in those patients with hypertension, diastolic BP was reduced without modification of their antihypertensive treatment.

In the HPS, there were 1,981 diabetics who had experienced a prior MI or other CHD event. These patients were treated with simvastatin (40 mg) or placebo in addition to other medications. As noted in **Figure 8.3**, a significant decrease in the occurrence of a new major vascular event was noted in the group of patients receiving the statin. In the 3,982 diabetics with no prior CHD history as well as in the total diabetics (with and without prior MI), a significant reduction in events was noted (**Figure 8.3**).

The Diabetes Atherosclerosis Intervention Study (DAIS) presented more positive evidence that correction of lipoprotein abnormalities in patients with type 2 diabetes can have an impact on the progression of coronary artery disease. Investigators found that fenofi-

FIGURE 8.2 — Effect of Pravastatin on Relative Risks of Cardiovascular Events in Patients With or Without Clinically Diagnosed Diabetes

End point Patient Number (N)	Placebo Nondiabetic (1774) Diabetic (304)	Pravastatin Nondiabetic (1779) Diabetic (282)	% Change in RR
CHD death	89 / 30	69 / 27	−24 / −3
Total MI	158 / 49	122 / 35	−25 / −23
CABG	163 / 44	127 / 29	−24 / −30
Stroke	54 / 24	35 / 19	−37 / −14
All end points	437 / 112	349 / 81	−23 / −25

● Nondiabetics
○ Diabetics

Relative Risk

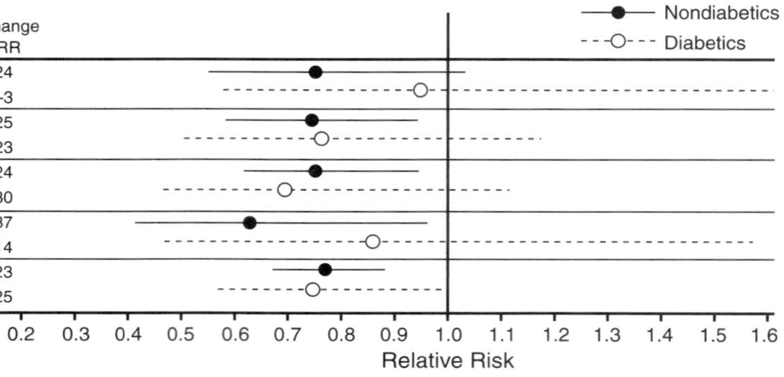

Abbreviations: CABG, coronary artery bypass grafting; CHD, coronary heart disease; MI, myocardial infarction; PTCA, percutaneous transluminal coronary angioplasty; RR, relative risk.

The numbers indicate patients with cardiovascular events. Relative risks for pravastatin compared with a placebo group are shown with 95% confidence intervals (CIs). Although a statistically significant decrease in CHD deaths, total MIs, and strokes was not noted in diabetic patients, the overall event rate (all end points) was decreased to an equivalent and significant degree in diabetic as well as nondiabetic patients.

Modified from: Goldberg RB, et al. *Circulation*. 1998;98:2513-2519.

FIGURE 8.3 — Effects of Simvastatin Therapy Compared With Placebo on First Major Vascular Event in Different Prior Disease Categories

Prior Disease Category	Simvastatin-Allocated Total Patients/ Incidence (%)	Placebo-Allocated Number/ Incidence (%)
Prior MI or Other CHD + Diabetes mellitus	325/972 (33.4%)	381/1009 (37.8%)
No Prior CHD + Diabetes mellitus	276/2006 (13.8%)	367/1976 (18.6%)
CHD or No Prior CHD + Diabetes mellitus	601/2978 (20.2%)	748/2985 (25.1%)

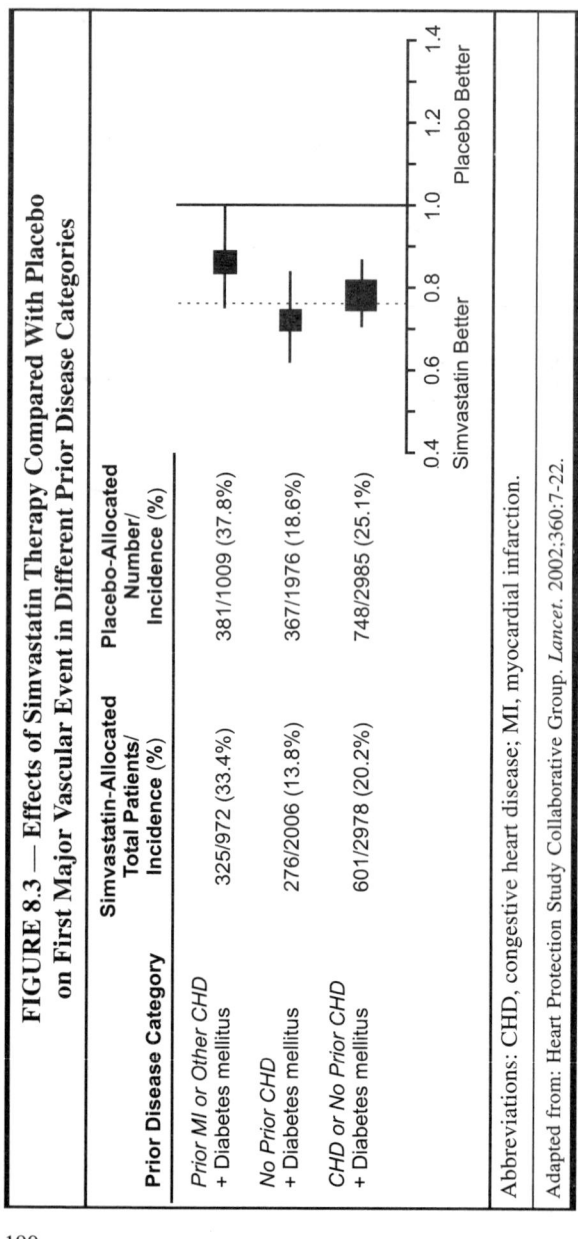

Abbreviations: CHD, congestive heart disease; MI, myocardial infarction.

Adapted from: Heart Protection Study Collaborative Group. *Lancet.* 2002;360:7-22.

brate therapy to normalize lipids reduced the progression of atherosclerosis by up to 40% in patients with type 2 diabetes.

DAIS was the first trial specifically designed to ascertain the effects of correcting lipoprotein abnormalities in people with type 2 diabetes. The 418 study subjects were followed for >3 years at 11 centers in Canada, Finland, France, and Sweden. All patients had lipid profiles typical of their condition: mild elevations of plasma triglycerides (mean, 214 mg/dL) and LDL (mean, 133 mg/dL), and a high ratio of total cholesterol to HDL (215 mg/dL/39 mg/dL = 5.5). Nearly half of the patients had a history of CHD, and a third had undergone a prior coronary intervention. At baseline, all subjects underwent coronary angiography to ensure that they had at least one measurable lesion. They were then randomized to micronized fenofibrate (200 mg/d) or placebo and followed for 3 years. Upon completion of treatment, all patients underwent coronary angiography to measure the progression of atherosclerosis.

Fenofibrate treatment was shown to reduce triglycerides, total cholesterol, and LDL, and to increase levels of HDL; notably, these results occurred in a population whose lipid levels were on average only slightly abnormal (**Figure 8.4**). In a subgroup of patients (one third of the total population)—with the most abnormal levels—triglycerides were reduced by 39%, LDL was reduced by 15%, and HDL was increased by 6.3%. In comparison with the placebo-treated group, patients treated with fenofibrate had a 40% reduction in the rate of progression of localized lesions. These changes were directly related to the lipid levels attained during the treatment period. CHD progression was reduced in both men and women, as well as in patients with and without a history of prior coronary interventions. There was also an accompanying 23% reduction in combined CHD events. Thus this study

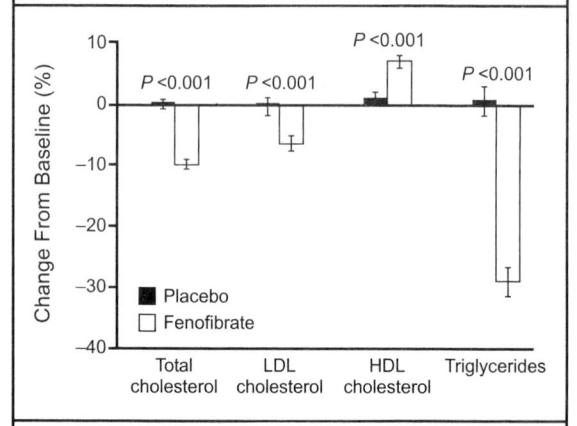

FIGURE 8.4 — Changes in Lipid Values From Baseline in Placebo and Fenofibrate Groups

Abbreviations: LDL, low-density lipoprotein; HDL, high-density lipoprotein.

Diabetes Atherosclerosis Intervention Study Investigators. Effect of fenofibrate on progression of coronary artery disease in type 2 diabetes: the Diabetes Atherosclerosis Intervention Study, a randomised study. *Lancet*. 2001;357:907.

provided good evidence that correcting (or even partially correcting) the lipid abnormalities in diabetic subjects is beneficial and that medication other than a statin can be effective.

Other studies have also demonstrated the metabolic benefits of fenofibrate alone and in combination with HMG-CoA reductase inhibitors in persons with low HDL levels and those with type 2 diabetes.

Therapy for Dyslipidemia in Diabetic Patients

Weight reduction and increased physical activity may lead to decreased triglycerides and increased HDL levels and also to a modest lowering of LDL cholesterol levels. Diabetic patients who are overweight should be given instructions on diet and increased physical activity. As noted, the proportion of saturated fat should be reduced. The American Diabetes Association (ADA) suggests an increase either in carbohydrate or in monounsaturated fat to compensate for the reduction in saturated fat (ie, cut down on fatty meats, butter, eggs, etc). Some (but not all) studies suggest that a high monounsaturated or polyunsaturated fat diet (more fish, olive oil, etc) may have better metabolic effects than a high-carbohydrate diet, although other experts have suggested that such a dietary modification may make weight loss more difficult in obese diabetic patients.

Recommendations of the American Heart Association for patients with CHD have suggested that adherence to a diet typically reduces LDL cholesterol by about 15-25 mg/dL. Thus if the LDL level exceeds the goal by >25 mg/dL (0.65 mmol/L) or if the patient is unlikely to follow the prescribed diet, the physician should probably institute pharmacologic therapy at the same time as behavioral therapy in high-risk patients (ie, diabetic patients) to achieve LDL levels <100 mg/dL. In other patients, dietary interventions may be evaluated at 6-week intervals with consideration of pharmacologic therapy after 3 and 6 months.

Treatment Goals for Lipoprotein Therapy

Because of frequent changes in glycemic control in diabetic patients and their effects on levels of lipoprotein levels, LDL, HDL, total cholesterol, and triglycerides should be measured every year in adult patients. If values decrease to goal levels (see below), assessment may be repeated every 2 years. In children with diabetes, consideration should be given to measuring lipoproteins after age 2 years, as suggested by the National Cholesterol Education Program (NCEP) Reports of the Expert Panel on Blood Cholesterol in Children and Adolescents. Optimal LDL cholesterol levels for adults with diabetes are <70 mg/dL (especially if there is evidence of CHD), optimal HDL cholesterol levels are >45 mg/dL, desirable triglyceride levels are <150 mg/dL, and desirable total cholesterol levels are <200 mg/dL. Nondiabetic women tend to have higher HDL cholesterol levels than men. It may be desirable to have even higher HDL cholesterol levels than 45 mg/dL. However, raising HDL cholesterol levels pharmacologically in diabetic patients is difficult since one of the effective agents for raising HDL levels is nicotinic acid, which, as noted, may actually raise blood glucose levels in diabetic patients. Fibrates may, however, raise HDL levels significantly without affecting glycemic control.

The recommendations for treatment of elevated LDL cholesterol generally follow the guidelines of both the NCEP and a recent ADA consensus development conference with the following caveats: Pharmacologic therapy should be initiated after behavioral interventions are tried. However, in patients with clinical CVD, pharmacologic therapy with a statin should be initiated at the same time that behavioral therapy is started.

In the context of the most recent NCEP report, it is suggested that diabetic subjects with clinical CHD and an LDL level >100 mg/dL (2.60 mmol/L) after medical nutrition therapy and glucose interventions be treated with pharmacologic agents. For diabetic patients without preexisting CHD, the current recommendations for starting pharmacologic therapy are an LDL level of ≥130 mg/dL (3.35 mmol/L), with a goal of ≥100 mg/dL (2.60 mmol/L) for LDL (diabetes should be considered a high CHD risk factor) (**Table 8.4**). These recommendations are based not only on the high

TABLE 8.4 — Guidelines for Lipid-Lowering Therapy in Patients With Diabetes

Other Conditions	Nutritional Therapy		Drug Therapy	
	Initiation Level	LDL Goal	Initiation Level	LDL Goal
With CHD or CVD	>100 mg/dL	≤100 mg/dL	>100 mg/dL	≤70 mg/dL
Without CHD or CVD	>100 mg/dL	≤100 mg/dL	≥130 mg/dL*	≤100 mg/dL

Abbreviations: CHD, coronary heart disease; CVD, cardiovascular disease; HDL, high-density lipoprotein; LDL, low-density lipoprotein.

* For diabetic patients with multiple CHD risk factors (low HDL [<35 mg/dL], hypertension, smoking, family history of CVD, or microalbuminuria or proteinuria), many authorities recommend initiation of drug therapy when levels are between 100 and 130 mg/dL.

incidence of CHD in patients with diabetes, but also on their higher case fatality rate once they have CHD. Since a large proportion of diabetic patients die from an acute coronary event before they reach the hospital, a preventive strategy based solely on secondary prevention after a CHD event would not be able to "save" large numbers of these diabetic patients. In patients with LDL levels >100 mg/dL, a variety of treatment strategies are available, including more aggressive diet therapy and pharmacologic treatment with a statin. In addition, if the HDL is <40 mg/dL, a fibric acid such as fenofibrate might be used in patients with an LDL between 100 and 129 mg/dL.

Lipid-Lowering Agents

A brief summary of the actions of the available agents for lipid lowering in patients with diabetes is shown in **Table 8.5**, along with the order of priority for treatment. Treatment of high LDL is considered as the first priority for pharmacologic therapy of dyslipidemia for a number of reasons. Clinical trials (4S, CARE, AFCAPS/TexCAPS, and HPS) have demonstrated the effectiveness of statins in reducing CHD in diabetic subjects. The Helsinki Heart Study, DAIS, and VA-HIT trials have indicated a reduction in CHD in this patient population with fibrate therapy. The effect of these pharmacologic agents on lipoproteins is summarized in **Table 8.6**. Generally, one or two agents are available in each class of drugs with the exception of the statins. The choice of a statin should depend principally on the LDL reduction needed to achieve the target (<100 mg/dL), the initial LDL level, and the judgment of the treating physician. The effects of the various statins in lower or moderate dosages on LDL, HDL, and triglycerides are summarized in **Table 8.7**.

TABLE 8.5 — Order of Priorities for Treatment of Diabetic Dyslipidemia in Adults

- LDL cholesterol lowering
  - Lifestyle interventions
  - Preferred: HMG CoA reductase inhibitor (statin)
  - Others: Bile acid–binding resin, cholesterol absorption inhibitor, fenofibrate, niacin, or combination therapy
- HDL cholesterol raising
  - Lifestyle interventions
  - Nicotinic acid or fibrates
- Triglyceride lowering
  - Lifestyle interventions
  - Glycemic control
  - Fibric acid derivative (gemfibrozil, fenofibrate), niacin, high-dose statins (in patients who also have high LDL cholesterol)
- Combined hyperlipidemia
  - First choice: improved glycemic control plus high-dose statin
  - Second choice: improved glycemic control plus statin plus fibric acid derivative
  - Third choice: Improved glycemic control plus statin plus nicotinic acid

Abbreviations: HDL, high-density lipoprotein; HMG CoA, 3-hydroxy-3-methylglutaryl coenzyme A; LDL, low-density lipoprotein.

Decision for treatment of high LDL before elevated triglyceride is based on clinical trial data indicating safety as well as efficacy of the available agents. The combination of statins with nicotinic acid, fenofibrate, and especially gemfibrozil may carry an increased risk of myositis. Patients with triglyceride levels >400 mg/dL require special consideration.

Adapted from: American Diabetes Association. *Diabetes Care*. 2004;27(suppl 1):S69.

TABLE 8.6 — Medications for the Treatment of Dyslipidemia in Adults

Agent	Effect on Lipoprotein			Clinical Trials in Diabetic Subjects
	LDL	HDL	Triglycerides	
First-Line Agents for Lowering LDL, Raising HDL, and Decreasing Triglycerides				
LDL-lowering HMG-CoA reductase inhibitor	↓↓	↔↑	↔↓	4S (simvastatin) CARE (pravastatin) CARDS (atorvastatin) HPS (simvastatin)
Fibric acid derivatives	↓↔↑	↑	↓↓	Helsinki (gemfibrozil) DAIS (fenofibrate) VA-HIT (gemfibrozil)
Second-Line Agents				
LDL-lowering bile acid–binding resins	↓	↔	↑	None
LDL- and triglyceride-lowering nicotinic acid*	↓	↑↑	↓↓	None

Abbreviations: CARDS, Collaborative Atorvastatin Diabetes Study; CARE, Cholesterol and Recurrent Events [trial]; DAIS, Diabetes Atherosclerosis Intervention Study; 4S, Scandinavian Simvastatin Survival Study; HDL, high-density lipoprotein; HMG-CoA, 3-hydroxy-3-methlglutaryl coenzyme A; HPS, Heart Protection Study; LDL, low-density lipoprotein; VA-HIT, Veterans Affairs High-Density Lipoprotein Intervention Trial.

* In diabetic patients, nicotinic acid should be restricted to ≤2 g/d; short-acting nicotinic acid is preferred.

TABLE 8.7 — Efficacy of HMG-CoA Reductase Inhibitors

Drug	Dose (mg/d)	% Δ in LDL-c	% Δ in HDL-c	% Δ in TG
Atorvastatin[1]	5	− 29	+ 8	− 25
	10	− 36	+ 7	− 13
	20	− 46	+ 6	− 22
	40	− 50	+ 3	− 30
	80	− 58	+ 2	− 26
Fluvastatin	20[2]	− 21	+ 3	− 8
	40[2]	− 26	+ 3	− 12
	80[3]*	− 32	—	—
	80[4]†	− 34	+ 8.5	− 12.4
Lovastatin[5]	20	− 24	+ 7	− 10
	40	− 34	+ 9	− 16
	80	− 40	+ 10	− 19
Pravastatin	10[6]	− 18	+ 5	− 5
	20[7]	− 25	+ 16	− 13
	40[8]	− 28	+ 7	− 11
	80[9]	− 37	+ 3	− 19
Rosuvastatin	5[10]	− 42	+ 8	− 16
	10[10]	− 47	+ 9	− 19
	20[11]	− 52	+ 10	− 20
	40[11]	− 57	+ 10	− 23
Simvastatin	5[12]	− 23	+ 8	− 10
	10[12]	− 28	+ 6	− 9
	20[12]	− 37	+ 6	− 12
	40[13]	− 40	+ 12	− 19
	80[13]	− 46	+ 4‡	− 19‡
	80[13]	− 46	+ 10§	− 36§

Abbreviations: HMG-CoA, 3-hydroxy-3-methylglutaryl coenzyme A; LDL-c, low-density lipoprotein cholesterol; HDL-c, high-density lipoprotein cholesterol; TG, triglyceride.

Continued

* Administered as 40 mg bid.
† Administered as 80-mg sustained-release tablet at bedtime.
‡ TG <200 mg/dL.
§ TG >200 mg/dL.

1. Data for 5 mg/d (n = 13) from Nawrocki JW et al. *Arterioscler Thromb Vasc Biol.* 1995;15:678-682. Data for 10 mg/d (n = 1090) from: (1) Bertolini S et al. *Atherosclerosis.* 1997;130:191-197; (2) Dart A et al. *Am J Cardiol.* 1997;80:39-44; (3) Davidson M et al. *Am J Cardiol.* 1997;79:1475-1481; (4) Heinonen TM et al. *Clin Ther.* 1996;18:853-863; and (5) Nawrocki JW et al. *Arterioscler Thromb Vasc Biol.* 1995;15:678-682. Data for 40 mg/d (n = 26) from: (1) Cilla DD et al. *J Clin Pharmacol.* 1996;36:604-609; and (2) Nawrocki JW et al. *Arterioscler Thromb Vasc Biol.* 1995;15:678-682. Data for 80 mg/d (n = 11) from Nawrocki JW, et al. *Arterioscler Thromb Vasc Biol.* 1995;15:678-682. Jones P et al. *Am J Cardiol.* 1998;81:582-587 contributes data for 10, 20, 40, and 80 mg/d.
2. Data for 20 mg/d (n = 1066) and 40 mg/d (n = 633) from a summary of blinded, placebo-controlled trials: Peters TK et al. *Drugs.* 1994;47(suppl 2):64-72.
3. Data from the largest single controlled study using this dose (n = 266): *Physicians' Desk Reference.* 54th ed. Montvale, NJ: Medical Economics Company, Inc; 2000:2021-2024.
4. Data from Olsson AG et al. *Clin Ther.* 2001;23:45-61.
5. Data from the EXCEL Study (n = 8245): Bradford RH et al. *Arch Intern Med.* 1991;151:43-49.
6. Data from a double-blind trial (n = 138): Steinhagen-Thiessen E. *Cardiology.* 1994;85:244-254.
7. Data from a double-blind trial (n = 303): The Lovastatin Pravastatin Study Group. *Am J Cardiol.* 1993;71: 810-815.
8. Data are taken as mean from three clinical trials with sample size of at least 500 each (CARE, WOSCOPS, and REGRESS).
9. Data from pooled analysis of two multicenter, double-blind, placebo-controlled studies, n = 277. Package insert for Pravachol. Bristol-Myers Squibb Co., Princeton, NJ, 2001.
10. Data from Jones PH et al. *Am J Cardiol.* 2003;92:152-160.
11. Data from Schneck EW et al. *Am J Cardiol.* 2003;91:33-41.
12. Data from: (1) Farmer JA et al. *Clin Ther.* 1992; 14:708-717; (2) Douste-Blazy P et al. *Drug Invest.* 1993;6:353-361; (3) Steinhagen-Thiessen E. *Cardiology.* 1994;85:244-254; (4) Lambrecht LJ, Malini PL. *Acta Cardiol.* 1993;48:541-554.
13. Data from Stein EA et al. *Am J Cardiol.* 1998;82: 311-316.

SELECTED READING

American Diabetes Association. Diabetes mellitus and exercise (position statement). *Diabetes Care*. 2001;24:S51-S55.

American Diabetes Association. Management of dyslipidemia in adults with diabetes (ADA recommendations). *Diabetes Care*. 2001;24(suppl 1):558-561.

American Diabetes Association. Nutrition recommendations and principles for people with diabetes mellitus (position statement). *Diabetes Care*. 2001;24:S44-S47.

Athyros VG, Papageorgiou AA, Athyrou VV, Demitriadis DS, Kontopoulos AG. Atorvastatin and micronized fenofibrate alone and in combination in type 2 diabetes with combined hyperlipidemia. *Diabetes Care*. 2002;25:1198-1202.

Colhoun HM, Betteridge DJ, Durrington PN, et al CARDS investigators. Primary prevention of cardiovascular disease with atorvastatin in type 2 diabetes in the Collaborative Atorvastatin Diabetes Study (CARDS): multicentre randomised placebo-controlled trial. *Lancet*. 2004;364:685-696.

Diabetes Atherosclerosis Intervention Study Investigators. Effect of fenofibrate on progression of coronary-artery disease in type 2 diabetes: the Diabetes Atherosclerosis Intervention study, a randomised study. *Lancet*. 2001;357:905-910.

Executive Summary of the Third Report of the National Cholesterol Education Program (NCEP) Expert Panel on Detection, Evaluation, and Treatment of High Blood Cholesterol in Adults (Adult Treatment Panel III). *JAMA*. 2001;285:2486-2497.

Goldberg RB, Mellies MJ, Sacks FM, et al. Cardiovascular events and their reduction with pravastatin in diabetic and glucose-intolerant myocardial infarction survivors with average cholesterol levels: subgroup analyses in the Cholesterol and Recurrent Events (CARE) trial. The Care Investigators. *Circulation*. 1998;98:2513-2519.

Grundy SM, Cleeman JI, Merz CN, et al; National Heart, Lung, and Blood Institute; American College of Cardiology Foundation; American Heart Association. Implications of recent clinical trials for the National Cholesterol Education Program Adult Treatment Panel III guidelines. *Circulation*. 2004;110:227-239.

Heart Protection Study Collaborative Group. MRC/BHF Heart Protection Study of cholesterol lowering with simvastatin in 20,536 high-risk individuals: a randomised placebo-controlled trial. *Lancet*. 2002;360:7-22.

Kirpichnikov D, Sowers JR. Effects of ACE inhibitor therapy on development of type 2 diabetes in hypertensive patients. *Cardiol Rev*. 2000;6:5-7.

Robins SJ. Targeting low high-density lipoprotein cholesterol for therapy: lessons from the Veterans Affairs High-Density Lipoprotein Intervention Trial. *Am J Cardiol*. 2001;88(suppl):19N-23N.

Rubins HB, Robins SJ, Collins D, et al. Gemfibrozil for the secondary prevention of coronary heart disease in men with low levels of high-density lipoprotein cholesterol. Veterans Affairs High-Density Lipoprotein Cholesterol Intervention Trial Study Group. *N Engl J Med*. 1999;341:410-418.

Sacks FM for the Expert Group on HDL Cholesterol. The role of high-density lipoprotein (HDL) cholesterol in the prevention and treatment of coronary heart disease: expert group recommendations. *Am J Cardiol*. 2002;90:139-143.

Saito I, Folsom AR, Brancati FL, Duncan BB, Chambless LE, McGovern PG. Nontraditional risk factors for coronary heart disease incidence among persons with diabetes: the Atherosclerosis Risk in Communities (ARIC) study. *Ann Intern Med*. 2000;133:81-91.

Sowers JR. Effects of statins on the vasculature: implications for aggressive lipid management in the cardiovascular metabolic syndrome. *Am J Cardiol*. 2003;91(suppl):14B-22B.

Velussi M, Cernigoi AM, Tortul C, Merni M. Atorvastatin for the management of type 2 diabetic patients with dyslipidemia. A midterm (9 months) treatment experience. *Diabetes Nutr Metab*. 1999;12:407-412.

9 Cardiovascular Risk Reduction: Antiplatelet Therapy

Because of the high risk of cardiovascular disease (CVD) in type 2 diabetics, most of these patients (including women) should receive aspirin if tolerated. According to an analysis by the Antiplatelet Trialists Collaboration, aspirin lowers the risk for myocardial infarction (MI) and appears to be effective for the secondary prevention of stroke. The major issue relates to dosing. In diabetes, there is markedly increased platelet aggregation/adhesion, endothelial cell adhesive properties, and vascular inflammation that likely require an aspirin dosage >81 mg daily.

The American Diabetes Association (ADA) has issued several sets of guidelines for aspirin therapy in adults with diabetes. The ADA recommends that in diabetic patients without specific contraindications, aspirin should be given for:
- Secondary prevention of cardiovascular (CV) events in both women and men with clinical evidence of macrovascular disease (stroke, transient ischemic attacks, MI, vascular bypass procedures)
- Primary prevention in adult diabetics who have one or more risk factors for CVD (hypertension, smoking, family history of coronary heart disease [CHD], obesity, dyslipidemia, or albuminuria) or are ≥30 years of age; in other words, in a large majority of diabetic patients.

The ADA indicates that the prophylactic use of aspirin has not been systemically studied in persons <30

years of age and that aspirin should not be recommended for those <21 years of age because of the risk of Reye's syndrome. Doses of enteric-coated aspirin 81 to 325 mg have been recommended. Contraindications cited by the ADA include:
- Allergies to aspirin
- Recent gastrointestinal bleeding
- Clinically active liver disease
- A known propensity to bleed.

The evidence supporting prophylactic aspirin use in adult diabetics is substantial. Three prospective trials in both men and women with diabetes, the Early Treatment Diabetic Retinopathy Study (ETDRS), the Hypertension Optimal Treatment (HOT) study, and the Heart Outcomes Prevention Evaluation (HOPE) study, showed benefits of aspirin therapy in the primary prevention of CVD, including MI. The HOT study results also reduced concerns about cerebrovascular bleeding as a complication of aspirin therapy. In patients in the HOT trial *whose hypertension was controlled*, the use of aspirin decreased the occurrence of MI. Although there is considerable evidence supporting the benefits of aspirin in primary prevention in diabetic patients, many diabetics may still not be taking aspirin despite the release of the ADA recommendations and the results of recent trials.

Although a number of antiplatelet agents are currently available, aspirin remains the most effective and least expensive platelet inhibitor. Beneficial effects of aspirin have been demonstrated in patients with diabetes, hypertension, and hypercholesterolemia as well as in people with evidence of CVD. It is unclear at present what is the lowest effective dose of aspirin in diabetic patients, but doses of 160 to 325 mg are most commonly recommended. These doses of aspirin, which are higher than the 81 mg/day recommended for the prevention of CV events in nondiabetics, may be required to counteract the enhanced endothelial adhesiveness and enhanced inflammation that occur in the vasculature of diabetic patients.

There are several new treatments that target platelet activity by inhibiting platelet adhesion and/or aggregation. Aspirin inhibits thromboxane A_2-mediated platelet adhesion. Two other agents, clopidogrel (Plavix) and ticlopidine (Ticlid), have an alternative mechanism of action; they block complementary pathways of platelet activation and aggregation. The different modes of action of these agents and aspirin provide the rationale for combination therapy. Antagonists to the platelet GPIIb/IIIa receptor can prevent fibrinogen binding and block the changes the receptor undergoes to enable it to mediate platelet aggregation. For diabetic patients who cannot tolerate aspirin, ticlopidine and clopidogrel may be used. They are relatively expensive but are otherwise reasonable alternative antiplatelet agents in diabetic patients.

SELECTED READING

American Diabetes Association. Aspirin therapy in diabetes. *Diabetes Care*. 2004;27(suppl 1):S72-S74.

Antiplatelet Trialists' Collaboration. Collaborative overview of random trials with antiplatelet therapy—I: Prevention of death, myocardial infarction, and stroke by prolonged antiplatelet therapy in various categories of patients. *BMJ*. 1994;308:81-106.

Hart RG, Halperin JL, McBride R, Benavente O, Man-Son-Hing M, Kronmal RA. Aspirin for the primary prevention of stroke and other major vascular events: meta-analysis and hypothesis. *Arch Neurol*. 2000;57:326-332.

Rolka DB, Fagot-Campagna A, Narayan KM. Aspirin use among adults with diabetes: estimates from the Third National Health and Nutrition Examination Survey. *Diabetes Care*. 2001;24:197-201.

10 Cardiovascular Risk Reduction: Control of Diabetes

Diabetes represents an increasingly common disease that may result in disabilities that decrease the quality of life and increase direct and indirect medical costs. Chronic complications accounted for >50% of the estimated $300 billion spent for care of patients with diabetes in the United States. It is becoming increasingly clear that these complications can be significantly reduced by aggressive treatment of risk factors such as hypertension and dyslipidemia in addition to hyperglycemia. Despite this knowledge, the level of care for people with diabetes is suboptimal, even in developed nations. Unfortunately, health policy makers and providers are frequently unaware of (or have failed to act upon) the considerable evidence supporting the role of lifestyle changes (ie, increase in physical activity and adhering to a healthy diet) in the primary prevention of type 2 diabetes or the therapeutic strategies to prevent or delay the complications of diabetes.

Both in patients with type 1 and type 2 diabetes, prospective studies have shown an association between the degree of hyperglycemia and increased risk of microvascular complications (ie, retinopathy, nephropathy), macrovascular events, myocardial infarction (MI), stroke, peripheral vascular disease, and all-cause mortality. The relative risk of MI seems to increase with any increase in glycemia to levels >100 mg/dL, whereas the risk for microvascular disease is thought to occur only with more extreme hyperglycemia. The Diabetes Control and Complications Trial (DCCT) showed an association between blood glucose levels

207

and the progression of microvascular complications in patients with type 1 diabetes for glycosylated hemoglobin (HbA_{1C}) over the range of 6% to 11% after a mean of 6 years of follow-up. In the United Kingdom Prospective Diabetes Study (UKPDS), a similar relationship was seen in patients with type 2 diabetes. Any reduction in HbA_{1C} reduced the risk of complications, with the lowest risk being in those with HbA_{1C} values in the normal range (<6.0%). Acceptable ranges and goals are given in **Table 10.1**.

Glycation refers to a linkage of carbohydrate to protein. This is an irreversible process in which glucose in the plasma attaches itself to the hemoglobin component of red blood cells. The life span of a red blood cell is 120 days. Therefore, glycated hemoglobin assays, one of which measures HbA_{1C}, reflect the average blood glucose concentration over this period of time. HbA_{1C} measurement depends on the percentage of hemoglobin molecules that have glucose attached (ie, about 5% is average).

Prevention of Type 2 Diabetes: Lifestyle and Drugs

A number of observational and interventional studies have shown that lifestyle intervention reduces the risk of developing type 2 diabetes mellitus. In a Swedish study in subjects with an increased risk for development of type 2 diabetes, lifestyle interventions decreased the development of diabetes over 5 years to 10.6% compared with 28.6% in a control group. Improvement in glucose tolerance and decreases in development of type 2 diabetes were related both to increased exercise and weight reduction; both contributed equally and independently to reduction in risk of diabetes.

Several other studies comparing diet, exercise, and diet plus exercise with a nontreatment control group

TABLE 10.1 — Glycemic Control in People With Diabetes*

	Normal	Goal
Whole blood values		
Average preprandial glucose[†]	<100 mg/dL	80-120 mg/dL
Average bedtime glucose[†]	<110 mg/dL	100-140 mg/dL
Plasma values		
Average preprandial glucose[‡]	<110 mg/dL	90-130 mg/dL
Average bedtime glucose[‡]	<120 mg/dL	110-150 mg/dL
HbA$_{1C}$	<6%	<7%

Abbreviation: HbA$_{1C}$, glycosylated hemoglobin.

* The values shown in this table are by necessity generalized to the entire population of individuals with diabetes. Patients with comorbid diseases or the very young and older adults may warrant different treatment goals. These values are for nonpregnant adults. HbA$_{1C}$ is referenced to a nondiabetic range of 4.0% to 6.0% (mean 5.0%).
[†] Measurement of capillary blood glucose.
[‡] Values calibrated to plasma glucose.

Modified from: American Diabetes Association. Clinical practice recommendations—2000. *Diabetes Care*. 2000;23(suppl 1):S33.

have reported that lifestyle approaches have reduced the occurrence of diabetes by 30% to 55% compared with control groups. The recently reported Diabetes Prevention Program (DPP) reported a 56% reduction in new-onset diabetes with lifestyle interventions in a population at high risk for development of this disease. In contrast, persons randomized to metformin treatment only had a 31% reduction in development of diabetes. This was a costly study and may not be practical given the increasing limitation of health care resources and poor reimbursement for preventive health care measures. It does, however, emphasize the importance of lifestyle modifications and what can be accomplished.

Diet

Dietary treatment is an essential component of management in patients with diabetes. The goals of nutritional intervention in patients with type 2 diabetes are to:

- Maintain near normal or normal blood glucose levels
- Attain and maintain a body weight as close to ideal body weight as possible
- Utilize a low-fat, high-fiber, low-sodium diet that promotes lipid and blood pressure (BP) lowering.

Traditional dietary recommendations emphasize reduction of both the total and saturated fat content and replacement with complex carbohydrates (ie, 50% to 55% of dietary calories). However, it must be kept in mind that in type 2 diabetic patients such diets may cause postprandial hyperglycemia. This can be moderated by smaller feedings and increased dietary fiber intake. Generally, a weight-reduction, heart-smart diet is appropriate for type 2 diabetics as these patients have a high risk for CVD.

General guidelines for nutritional approaches to patients with diabetes have been developed that take into consideration the heterogeneity of patients with type 2 diabetes (**Table 10.2**). The dietary approach should be monitored not only on the basis of body weight, but also on the impact on metabolic parameters, BP, and the quality of life. In general, this type of diet can be tolerated without difficulty and should include nutritional foods and foods that are high in calcium, potassium, and magnesium.

More than 75% of people with type 2 diabetes are obese; their weight loss is a primary intervention goal. Caloric restriction improves glucose control and the loss of as little as 5% of body weight improves insulin sensitivity, reduces insulin secretion, and decreases hepatic glucose production. Weight reduction is best accomplished by a combination of modest caloric restriction and physical activity. Initial or sustained weight reduction is difficult without some increase in physical activity. Increased aerobic activity, in turn, has a direct beneficial effect on insulin sensitivity/glucose utilization and may also lower BP and increase HDL cholesterol levels.

An approach to weight reduction should be realistic, with weight loss of one half to one pound per week being recommended. Generally, a decrease of 500 calories/day is needed to produce a 1-lb loss of weight per week. Substantial weight loss is difficult and many patients will fail to lose weight and keep it down on the first or second try. Having diabetes should be a motivating factor. All patients should be advised to avoid fad diets (ie, diets of the month, high-fat, or high-protein miracle diets). These may work for a short period of time but have not been shown to produce long-term weight loss. The current "low-carb" diet fad has led to dramatic changes in the eating habits of millions of Americans. There is little doubt that such diets will result in weight loss because they basically

TABLE 10.2 — Nutrition Goals, Principles, and Recommendations*

- Calories—Sufficient to attain and/or maintain a reasonable body weight for adults, normal growth and development for children and adolescents, and adequate nutrition through pregnancy and lactation
- Protein:
  - 10% to 20% of daily calories
  - No more than adult recommended daily allowance (RDA) (0.8 g/kg body weight per day) with evidence of nephropathy (ie, if 2000 cal/d, about 200-400 cal/d of protein; since 1 g protein = 4 cal, then about 50 g = 200 cal/d of protein)
- Fat:
  - *Saturated* fat <7% to 10% (or about 140-200 cal/d of fat on a 2000 cal/d diet (1 g fat = 9 cal); 15-22 g of fat per day (ie, $9 \times 20 = 180$ cal/d)
  - Polyunsaturated fat up to 10% of total calories (about 200 cal/d on a 2000 cal/d diet)
  - Total fat varies with treatment goals; generally <25% of total calories
  - Predominantly monounsaturated fat
- Cholesterol <250 mg/d
- Carbohydrate:
  - Difference after protein and fat goals have been met
  - Percentage varies with treatment goals
- Sweeteners:
  - Sucrose (ie, table sugar [cane or beet]) need not be restricted; must be substituted as carbohydrate
  - Nutritive sweeteners have no advantage over sucrose and must be substituted as carbohydrate
  - Nonnutritive sweeteners (ie, saccharin, aspartame, acesulfame potassium, and sucralose) approved by the Food and Drug Administration (FDA) are safe to consume
- Fiber 20-35 g/d (All-Bran, rye bread, etc)
- Sodium <2400 mg/d
- Alcohol—moderate usage, ie, less than two alcoholic beverages daily
- Vitamins and minerals—same as the general population

Goals must always be individualized.

* It is important to check food labels for exact amount of each component.

lower calorie intake. The weight loss over the first week is accounted for mainly by a loss of fluid. The long-term safety of these diets is questionable, as are the long-term very low-carb, high-protein diets.

If the first miracle diet had worked, there would be no need for a new one every 3 to 6 months. Getting the diabetic patient on a sensible regimen for weight loss is an important step in management and, at the present time, the guidelines noted in **Table 10.2** seem reasonable. More detailed information about diet and diabetes can be found in the numerous publications of the American Diabetes Association or in standard textbooks on diabetes.

Exercise

Both obesity and inactivity contribute significantly to the development of type 2 diabetes. Regular aerobic exercise may delay or prevent type 2 diabetes, and it also helps in therapy of patients with diabetes. Regular aerobic exercise in type 2 diabetic patients helps to:
- Enhance a weight-reduction program
- Improve glycemic control
- Reduce BP and improve the lipid profile
- Enhance quality of life and psychological well-being
- Reduce the requirements for oral antidiabetic agents or insulin.

Exercise, particularly the aerobic variety that includes walking or motion exercise, is beneficial in type 2 diabetes as it helps maintenance of weight reduction and improves insulin sensitivity. Mechanisms by which aerobic exercise improves insulin sensitivity include decreases in intra-abdominal fat, increases in insulin-sensitive skeletal muscle fibers, and reduction in free fatty acids that interfere with insulin action. In addition, exercise provides the additional benefits of possibly lowering BP, improving cardiovascular function, raising HDL, and lowering triglycerides.

There are several caveats that should be considered in recommending exercise in type 2 diabetic patients. Because many type 2 patients are obese and have led sedentary lives, they are often in poor physical condition. A thorough history and physical examination and an electrocardiogram (ECG) should generally be performed before these patients engage in exercise. Lower levels of exercise should be initiated and resistance training (ie, weight lifting) should be done with caution (lifting of 5- to 10-lb weights can probably be undertaken without concern). If an individual does plan to engage in heavier weight lifting or vigorous exercise (ie, running), he or she should probably have an exercise stress test and a careful ophthalmologic examination to avoid exacerbation of retinopathy. Strenuous exercise is contraindicated in diabetic patients with active proliferative retinopathy, significant neuropathy, or cardiovascular disease (CVD). Peripheral neuropathy involving decreased sensitivity in the soles of the feet and inadequate peripheral pulses preclude running or jogging. In diabetics who exercise, it is important that they have comfortable shoes with appropriate arch supports. Appropriate precautions for diabetic patients with medical complications are given in **Table 10.3**.

Most diabetic patients can undertake a program of walking. Biking and swimming are often safe and useful exercises in patients with neuropathy where foot placement and gait may be compromised. Generally, diabetic persons should begin slowly, exercise at regular intervals at least 3 to 4 times a week, and gradually increase the duration and intensity of their exercise program. Flexibility stretching is important to promote range of motion and prevent muscle and joint injury;

TABLE 10.3 — Precautions for Diabetic Patients With Medical Complications

- Insensitive feet or peripheral vascular insufficiency:
  - Avoid running
  - Choose walking, cycling, or swimming
  - Emphasize proper footwear
- Untreated or recently treated proliferative retinopathy; avoid exercises associated with:
  - Increased intra-abdominal pressure (ie, heavy weight lifting)
  - Valsalvalike maneuvers
  - Rapid head movements
  - Possible eye trauma
- Hypertension:
  - Avoid heavy lifting
  - Avoid Valsalvalike maneuvers

this is especially important in the elderly diabetic. There is no reason why diabetic patients cannot participate in sports such as golf or tennis. Limitations should include chest or leg pain (intermittent claudication). Finally, armchair exercises can be performed by those patients confined to a wheelchair or those with very limited mobility. A diet and exercise program is useful not only in helping with glucose control but also may favorably impact lipid and BP abnormalities.

One potential problem associated with any aerobic exercise program is hypoglycemia in patients receiving oral antidiabetic agents or insulin. Hypoglycemia can occur during or as long as 12 to 18 hours after aerobic exercise. Monitoring of blood glucose is useful in adjusting oral medications or insulin to prevent exercise-induced hypoglycemia. Timing of exercise is important in the diabetic patient. Exercise performed between 3 PM and 5 PM may reduce nighttime hepatic glucose production and thus decrease fasting blood glucose levels. In addition, exercise after eating may reduce the postprandial hyperglycemia that often occurs in type 2 diabetes and which is increasingly associated with microvascular and macrovascular complications. The benefits of aerobic exercise in type 2 diabetic patients are achieved with exercise at least 3 times per week or every other day. Weight reduction is enhanced by exercise sessions carried out 5 to 6 times weekly (**Table 10.4**).

TABLE 10.4 — Guidelines for Safe Exercise

- At all times, patients should carry an identification card and wear a bracelet, necklace, or tag that identifies them as having diabetes
- If insulin is used:
  - Avoid exercise during peak insulin action
  - Administer insulin away from working limbs
- If the patient takes a single daily dose of intermediate-acting insulin, decrease the dose by as much as 30% to 35% before exercise
- If a combination of short- and intermediate-acting insulin is being given, decrease or omit the short-acting insulin by up to one third on days when exercise is planned. This may produce hyperglycemia later in the day that requires a second injection of short-acting insulin
- If only short-acting insulin is being used, reduce the preexercise dose and reduce the postexercise dose based on self-monitoring of blood glucose. The total dose may need to be reduced by as much as 30% to 50% on days when exercise is planned.
- Be alert for signs of hypoglycemia during and for several hours after exercise. Have immediate access to a source of readily absorbable carbohydrate (such as glucose tablets) to treat hypoglycemia
- Take sufficient fluids before, after, and if necessary, during exercise to prevent dehydration

Diabetic Retinopathy

The importance of regular ophthalmologic evaluations and early detection and treatment of visual problems in diabetic persons cannot be overemphasized. More than 5000 cases of blindness related to diabetes occur in the United States yearly. Diabetes is the leading cause of new blindness in Americans between the ages of 20 and 74 years. Over 60% of patients with type 2 diabetes have some form of diabetic retinopathy 20 years after the diagnosis is made. Loss of vision associated with proliferative retinopathy and macular edema can be reduced by 50% with laser photocoagulation if identified in time.

This is the therapy of choice in those who have proliferative retinopathy; it reduces the risk of sudden and/or severe visual loss by up to 60%. The intent of photocoagulation is to stop neovascularization before recurrent hemorrhages into the vitreous cause irreversible visual loss. On occasions when retinal detachment and massive vitreous hemorrhage occur, closed vitrectomy can be performed to remove blood vitreous and fibrous tissue. In at least half of the cases, vision can be restored by this procedure.

Diabetic retinopathy, either in the form of macular edema or proliferative retinopathy, does not typically cause visual problems until a relatively advanced stage has been reached. Management results are better when the disease is diagnosed early and, accordingly, a yearly ophthalmologic examination by an ophthalmologist or optometrist experienced in diagnosing diabetic retinopathy is important.

Control of metabolic abnormalities and BP is important in the prevention and lessening of progression of both background (nonproliferative) and proliferative retinopathy.

Prevention of Lower-Extremity Peripheral Vascular Complications

Over 50% of nontraumatic amputations in the United States occur in diabetics, and it has been estimated that more than half of these amputations could have been prevented with proper foot care and control of abnormal glucose metabolism. Foot lesions leading to nontraumatic amputations are the result of peripheral vascular disease, polyneuropathy, and superimposed infections. The sudden development of a painful foot or ankle lesion, usually secondary to some trauma or irritation, often indicates that there is underlying vascular disease, which is clinically indicated by decreased or absent pulses, dependent rubor, and pallor on leg elevation (**Table 10.5**). The degree of vascular disease and its potential for treatment by surgical intervention can be determined by Doppler ultrasonography followed up with angiography. Revascularization procedures, such as bypass or angioplasty, may be helpful in treating patients for nonhealing lesions, claudication, or the healing of amputation suture/incision sites. On the other hand, these procedures are sometimes ineffective because of the diffuse nature of vascular lesions in diabetic patients. Smoking cessation is extremely important in the prevention of peripheral vascular disease and its progression in diabetic persons. Proper foot care and measures to slow down vascular injury (ie, glycemic control, management of lipids, platelet disorders, and normalization of BP) are important in preventing peripheral vascular disease in diabetics.

Pharmacologic Therapy

Pharmacologic therapy should be instituted in conjunction with diet and exercise. Agents currently available for type 2 diabetics if dietary and exercise pro-

TABLE 10.5 — Warning Symptoms and Signs of Diabetic Foot Problems

Cause	Symptoms	Signs
Vascular	Cold feet; intermittent claudication involving calf or foot; pain at rest, especially nocturnal, relieved by dependency	Absent pedal, popliteal, or femoral pulses; femoral bruits; dependent rubor, plantar pallor on elevation; prolonged capillary filling time (>3-4 sec); decreased skin temperature
Neurologic	*Sensory:* burning, tingling, or crawling sensations; pain and hypersensitivity; cold feet *Motor:* weakness (foot drop) *Autonomic:* diminished sweating	*Sensory:* deficits (vibratory, then pain and temperature perception), hyperesthesia *Motor:* diminished to absent deep tendon reflexes (↓ Achilles, then patellar reflexes); weakness *Autonomic:* diminished-to-absent sweating
Musculoskeletal	Gradual changes in foot shape, sudden painless change in foot shape, with swelling, without history of trauma	Cavus feet with claw toes; drop foot; "rocker-bottom" foot (Charcot's joint); neuropathic arthropathy
Dermatologic	Painful wounds; slow-healing or nonhealing wounds or necrosis; skin color changes (cyanosis, redness); chronic scaling, itching, or dry feet; recurrent infections (paronychia, athlete's foot)	*Skin:* abnormal dryness; chronic tinea infections; keratotic lesions with or without hemorrhage (plantar or digital); trophic ulcer *Hair:* diminished or absent *Nails:* trophic changes; onychomycosis; sublingual ulceration or abscess; ingrown nails with paronychia

grams are ineffective in reducing blood glucose and HbA_{1C} levels to a normal range include sulfonylureas and related compounds, biguanides, thiazolidinediones, α-glucosidase inhibitors, and insulin (**Table 10.6**). A rational approach in using available agents involves using those drugs particularly suited to the stage and extent of the disease, and progressing to combination therapy, which is eventually necessary in most patients (**Figure 10.1**).

■ Agents That Enhance Insulin Secretion
Sulfonylureas

Sulfonylureas, such as tolbutamide (Orinase) and tolazamide (Tolinase), and the newer preparations, such as glipizide (Glucotrol, Glucotrol XL) and glimepiride (Amaryl), were the first of the oral hypoglycemic agents. Their primary action is to enhance insulin secretion. Because they can increase insulin secretion at all glucose levels, they may cause hypoglycemia. All sulfonylureas bind to the β-cell of the pancreas and close ATP-sensitive potassium channels. As a result, calcium channels open, leading to an increase in cytoplasmic calcium, thus stimulating insulin secretion. One of these agents, glimepiride (Amaryl), appears to exert relatively selective inhibition of the ATP-sensitive potassium channel on the β-cell of the pancreas, having little or no effect on the vascular or cardiac ATP-sensitive potassium channels. This means that this agent may not impair preischemic reconditioning in the heart.

To a lesser extent than for insulin therapy, sulfonylureas, through resultant hyperinsulinemia, may cause weight gain as well as development of hypoglycemia. Some data suggests that the use of long-acting glipizide (Glucotrol XL) may result in less weight gain and, in addition, offers sustained glucose control over 24 hours. The kidney is important in the clearance of most sulfonylureas. Therefore, these agents should be used with caution in persons with impaired renal function. Sulfonylureas should also be used with caution in persons with impaired liver function. The concern that sulfonylureas directly increase CVD mortality (originally raised by the University Group Diabetes Project) has been largely allayed by the United Kingdom Prospective Diabetes Study (UKPDS). The UKPDS demonstrated that in the presence of a comparable degree of glycemic control, mortality did not differ in patients treated with either insulin or sulfonylureas. Sulfonylureas are generally appropriate drugs in patients with relative insulin deficiency. Such patients would typically be lean, with lower basal and postprandial insulin levels. In addition, based on the recent UKPDS, these patients tend to be younger (<46 years of age) and more likely to require insulin. Dosage and frequency of administration are listed in **Table 10.6**.

Repaglinide (Prandin)

Repaglinide is a nonsulfonylurea secretagogue of the meglitinide class. It binds to a nonsulfonylurea β-cell receptor and stimulates insulin secretion by inhibiting the ATP-sensitive potassium channel. It has rapid onset and offset of action and, therefore, needs to be taken with meals. It decreases the postprandial glycemic increase and may cause less weight gain and hypoglycemia than sulfonylureas. Repaglinide is primarily excreted in the feces, with little or no excretion by the kidney. Therefore, it can be used in individuals with impaired renal function. Since it is metabolized by the liver, it should not be used in patients with hepatic dysfunction. As with sulfonylureas, repaglinide shows an added benefit when given with metformin.

Nateglinide (Starlix)

Nateglinide is an N-acylphenylalanine derivative that acts by inhibiting the same ATP-sensitive potassium channel that is inhibited by sulfonylureas. It also

TABLE 10.6 — Characteristics of Currently Available Oral Antidiabetic Agents

Generic Name	Trade Name	Recommended Starting Dosage (mg)	Recommended Maximum Dosage (mg)	Duration of Action (h)
SULFONYLUREAS*				
First Generation				
Acetohexamide	Dymelor	125 bid	750 bid	10-14
Chlorpropamide	Diabinese	250 qd	500 qd	60
Tolazamide	Tolinase	100 qd	500 bid	12-24
Tolbutamide	Orinase	250 bid	1000 tid	6-12
Second Generation				
Glimepiride	Amaryl	1-2 qd	8 qd	24
Glipizide	Glucotrol	5 qd	20 bid	12-24
Glipizide (extended release)	Glucotrol XL	5 qd	20 qd	24
Glyburide	DiaBeta, Micronase	2.5-5 qd	10 bid	16-24
	Glynase PresTab	1.5-3 qd	6 bid	12-24

GLINIDES				
Meglitinide[†]				
Repaglinide	Prandin	0.5 bid-qid w/meals	4 qid w/meals	2-4
D-*Phenylalanine Derivative*[‡]				
Nateglinide	Starlix	120 tid w/meals	120 tid w/meals	2-4
THIAZOLIDINEDIONES[†]				
Pioglitazone	Actos	15-30 qd	45 qd	Plasma elimination half-life 3-7 h
Rosiglitazone	Avandia	2-4 qd	8 qd or 4 bid	Plasma elimination half-life 3-4 h
BIGUANIDE[§]				
Metformin	Glucophage	500 with dinner	2550	Plasma elimination half-life ≈6.2 h
	Glucophage XR	500 qd	2000	Plasma elimination half-life ≈24 h
ALPHA-GLUCOSIDASE INHIBITORS[§]				
Acarbose	Precose	25 tid w/meals	100 tid w/meals	Not absorbed systemically
Miglitol	Glyset	25 tid w/meals	50 tid w/meals	

Continued

Generic Name	Trade Name	Recommended Starting Dosage (mg)	Recommended Maximum Dosage (mg)	Duration of Action (h)
SULFONYLUREA/BIGUANIDE COMBINATION AGENTS				
Glipizide/metformin	Metaglip	2.5/250 qd w/meals	20/2000 qd w/meals	24
Glyburide/metformin	Glucovance	1.25/250 qd w/meals	2.5/500 qd w/meals	Plasma elimination half-life $\approx$ 10 h
THIAZOLIDINEDIONE/BIGUANIDE COMBINATION AGENT				
Rosiglitazone/metformin	Avandamet	2/500 bid w/meals	8/2000 qd w/meals	24

* Starting dosage for elderly and lean adults with diabetes may need to be reduced by up to 50%.
† Selection of initial dose depends on the patient's glucose level.
‡ Starting dosage may be reduced by 50% when patients are near the HbA_{1C} goal.
§ The dosage of metformin, acarbose, and miglitol must be titrated slowly to limit gastrointestinal side effects.

Modified from: *Physicians' Desk Reference*, 59th ed. Montvale, NJ: Thomson PDR; 2005.

has a rapid onset and offset of action and, therefore, needs to be taken with each meal. Nateglinide, like repaglinide, is metabolized to inactive metabolites by the liver and excreted in the feces. There is little or no excretion by the kidney.

■ Agents That Alter Insulin Action
Metformin (Glucophage)

Glucose lowering by this drug occurs primarily by decreasing hepatic glucose production, and to a lesser extent, by decreasing peripheral insulin resistance. Metformin acts by causing the translocation of glucose transporters from the microsomal fraction to the plasma membrane of hepatic and skeletal muscle cells. It does not stimulate insulin release and does not cause hypoglycemia. Moreover, it does not cause weight gain, and it improves the lipid profile by causing a decline in total and very low-density lipoprotein, triglycerides, total cholesterol, and LDL cholesterol, and an increase in HDL cholesterol. It is best suited for obese patients with type 2 diabetes who are unresponsive to diet alone and who are assumed to be insulin resistant. It has some anorectic properties and causes less weight gain than other oral agents or insulin. It is effective as monotherapy or in combination with other agents, such as insulin or insulin secretagogues, other insulin-sensitizing drugs, or inhibitors of glucose absorption such as acarbose. Results of studies have shown that the addition of nateglinide to metformin improved glycemic control in patients on metformin monotherapy who have failed to achieve HbA_{1C} goals.

The major risk of this drug, lactic acidosis, occurs with a frequency of 1:120,000 patient-year. Its major route of excretion is through the kidneys. Metformin is contraindicated in those with renal disease (creatinine ≥1.5 in males; ≥1.4 in females), in the presence of hepatic disease, and in patients with tis-

FIGURE 10.1 — Treatment Algorithm for Glycemic Control of Type 2 Diabetes

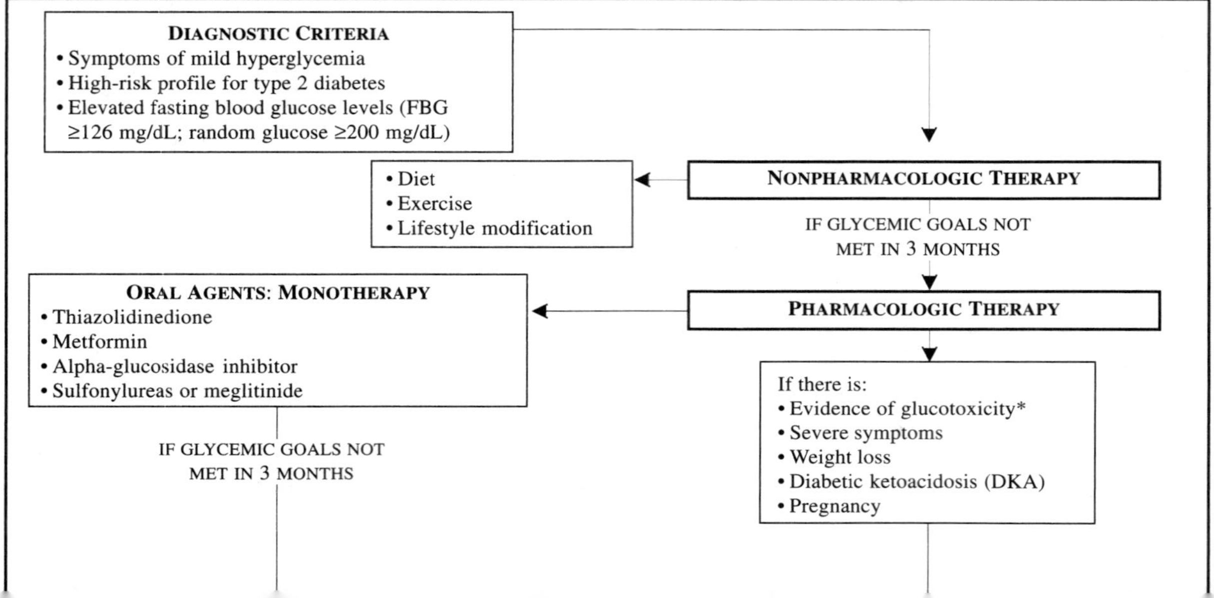

DIAGNOSTIC CRITERIA
- Symptoms of mild hyperglycemia
- High-risk profile for type 2 diabetes
- Elevated fasting blood glucose levels (FBG ≥126 mg/dL; random glucose ≥200 mg/dL)

NONPHARMACOLOGIC THERAPY
- Diet
- Exercise
- Lifestyle modification

IF GLYCEMIC GOALS NOT MET IN 3 MONTHS

PHARMACOLOGIC THERAPY

If there is:
- Evidence of glucotoxicity*
- Severe symptoms
- Weight loss
- Diabetic ketoacidosis (DKA)
- Pregnancy

ORAL AGENTS: MONOTHERAPY
- Thiazolidinedione
- Metformin
- Alpha-glucosidase inhibitor
- Sulfonylureas or meglitinide

IF GLYCEMIC GOALS NOT MET IN 3 MONTHS

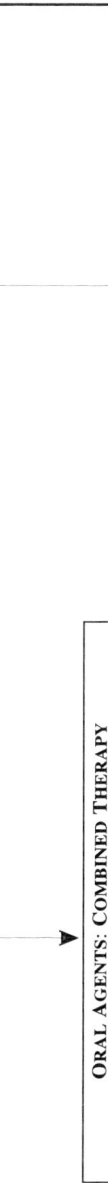

ORAL AGENTS: COMBINED THERAPY

- Thiazolidinedione + metformin
- Thiazolidinedione + (sulfonylurea/repaglinide)
- Alpha-glucosidase inhibitor + (sulfonylurea/repaglinide)
- Metformin + (sulfonylurea/repaglinide)
- Any combination is feasible, including drugs in triple combination[†]

OR

COMBINED: INSULIN + ORAL AGENT

- Single bedtime intermediate-acting insulin (adjusted to reduce FBG to <140 mg/dL consistently) plus daytime oral agent(s)

IF DAYTIME GLYCEMIC CONTROL NOT ACHIEVED IN 3 MONTHS, DISCONTINUE OR ADD/CHANGE ORAL AGENT

INSULIN ALONE[‡]

- Split-mixed regimen: intermediate- and fast-acting (70/30, 75/25), prebreakfast and predinner
- Multiple injections (3 or more) ± long-acting insulin
- Continuous subcutaneous insulin infusion (CSII)

IF HYPERGLYCEMIA INADEQUATELY CONTROLLED (HbA$_{1C}$ >8.5%) AND USING >30–75 U/DAY INSULIN

ADD THIAZOLIDINEDIONE OR METFORMIN OR ALPHA-GLUCOSIDASE INHIBITOR, EXCEPT WITH DKA AND PREGNANCY

---

* Insulin use may be temporary to reduce glucotoxicity; patient then may respond to sulfonylureas and other oral agents, alone or in combination.

† Many combinations not yet FDA-approved indication.

‡ Choice of insulin regimen based on individual assessment.

sue ischemia. In addition, the drug should be withheld for 48 hours after intravenous contrast administration.

Thiazolidinediones (Avandia, Actos)

These drugs appear to act by binding to a receptors that influence the differentiation of fibroblasts into adipocytes; free fatty acid levels are lowered. Clinically, their major effect is to decrease insulin resistance; this requires the presence of insulin to exert beneficial effects. In contrast to sulfonylureas and metformin, the effects of the thiazolidinediones may be progressive over time, and their full hypoglycemic effects may not be achieved until after 10 weeks of therapy. An elevated C peptide and being overweight may help to predict a beneficial response to these drugs as well as to metformin. These drugs are also usually synergistic with metformin in improving glucose control. Moreover, as insulin resistance is often accompanied by relative insulin deficiency, either a thiazolidinedione or metformin is often most effective when either or both drugs are given along with insulin or an insulin secretagogue.

The thiazolidinediones approved by the Food and Drug Administration (FDA) are rosiglitazone (Avandia) and pioglitazone (Actos). Both drugs cause some weight gain and increased adiposity. However, the increase in body fat may be associated with a shift from visceral to subcutaneous fat. This class of drugs can cause water retention and hemodilution. Therefore, they are not recommended for use in persons with stage 3 and 4 heart failure, and should be used with caution in anyone with cardiac dysfunction. Since they are metabolized by the liver, they should not be used in patients with hepatic dysfunction. It is recommended that liver enzymes be checked prior to the initiation of therapy with these agents and periodically thereafter.

■ Agents That Delay the Absorption of Carbohydrates
Alpha-Glucosidase Inhibitors (Precose, Glyset)

Alpha-glucosidase inhibitors include acarbose (Precose) and miglitol (Glyset). These agents inhibit the enzymatic degradation of sucrose, maltose, and other oligosaccharides. Thus they delay the absorption of carbohydrates and thereby lower the increase in postprandial blood glucose. The glucose-lowering effects of these drugs is proportional to the carbohydrate content of the diet. Both drugs must be taken with meals. Side effects are primarily gastrointestinal. Disaccharides not absorbed in the small intestine as a result of the action of these drugs enter the large intestine, where they are metabolized by bacteria to short-chain fatty acids. This may result in abdominal bloating, flatulence, and diarrhea that may be minimized by slowly titrating the dose of these drugs. Although alpha-glucosidase inhibitors do not cause hypoglycemia when used alone, they may increase the risk of hypoglycemia when combined with insulin or insulin secretagogue therapy such as the sulfonylureas. Although poorly absorbed, renal impairment can lead to an increase in plasma levels of these medications. Therefore they should not be used in patients with renal impairment.

Insulin

Insulin therapy is indicated in the treatment of all type 1 patients and in type 2 patients for initial therapy of severe hyperglycemia, after failure of oral agents, during perioperative periods, during and following an MI, or other acute hyperglycemic states. Insulin has been used in various combinations in type 2 diabetics, and new insulin analogues are becoming available for clinical use. The first available insulin analog was lispro insulin, representing a two–amino acid modification of regular insulin. Lispro insulin does not form aggregates following subcutaneous injection, allowing it to have a more rapid onset and a shorter duration of action. These properties may help minimize the postprandial rise in glucose and decrease the risk of late hypoglycemia. Any insulin therapy can, however, result in a weight gain and a tendency to develop hypoglycemia. The results of the UKPDS do not support the notion that exogenous insulin increases the risk of CVD. Insulin is often used in conjunction with sensitizing agents, but this combination can lead to significant weight gain (especially the combination of insulin and thiazolidinediones (such as Avandia or Actos). Ultimately, insulin therapy may become necessary in many patients with type 2 diabetes as pancreatic β-cell failure ensues. The addition of bedtime insulin to sulfonylureas and sensitizing agents may delay β-cell failure. Finally, it is appropriate to use insulin therapy during hospitalization for myocardial ischemia, stroke, and perioperative procedures if blood glucose levels are high. It is also important to maintain good glycemic control and avoid hypoglycemia (blood sugar <80-100 mg/dL) during hospitalization.

Details regarding types of insulin available and more specific regimens for use can be found in standard books on diabetes.

Use of Mineral Supplements

Certain mineral compounds, such as chromium picolinate, have been found, both in animal and human studies, to increase the effects of insulin in clearing blood glucose and increasing glycogen deposition in muscles. Studies are ongoing to determine the role of these compounds as adjuncts in the treatment of diabetes.

Glycemic Control: Does It Reduce Cardiovascular Events?

The Diabetes Control and Complications Trial provided unequivocal evidence of substantive reductions in chronic microvascular complications (retinopathy, nephropathy, and neuropathy) in a group of type 1 diabetic patients in whom intensive therapy maintained glucose at near normal levels over a 6-year period with a mean HbA_{1C} slightly above 7% compared with 9% in controls. The UKPDS also showed a significant risk reduction for microvascular events. However, the results of the UKPDS also demonstrated that rigorous glycemic control was difficult. For example, median HbA_{1C} concentrations 10 years after the study was initiated were higher than baseline values in patients assigned to intensive treatment. This inability to tightly control glucose may have accounted, in part, for the findings of greater benefit of BP lowering compared to tight glucose control. For example, there were substantial reductions in any end points related to diabetes (24%), deaths related to diabetes (32%), and microvascular disease (37%) in those achieving tight control of BP. In contrast, improvements in end points with tight glycemic control were not as great: reduction of end points related to diabetes (only 10%), and microvascular disease (25%). There were no significant benefits in either stroke or heart failure reduction in those in the intensive glucose-lowering group compared with a 44% decrease in stroke and a 56% decrease in heart failure in the group assigned to tight BP control.

The overall results of the UKPDS can be subdivided into two components:
- Results in patients randomized to insulin and to sulfonylurea agents (glyburide or chlorpropamide (n = 2729)

- Results achieved in overweight patients randomized to metformin therapy (n = 342).

Both treatment cohorts were compared with patients who were treated less intensively initially with diet alone. By the end of the study, however, many patients in the diet-alone group required some form of medication for treatment of hyperglycemia. Findings from the sulfonylurea and/or insulin arm of the study showed that the risk of one diabetes-related end point was reduced by 12% and microvascular events were reduced by 25% compared with the diet-alone group. The results may actually have been better in the intensively treated group compared with the diet-only group if fewer patients in the latter group had crossed over to specific therapy.

In the UKPDS study, both sulfonylureas and insulin were associated with a greater weight gain as well as more hypoglycemic episodes than metformin. Further, treatment with the latter agent resulted in a greater improvement in outcome than with sulfonylurea/insulin treatment. Patients treated with metformin as first-line therapy had a decrease in diabetes-related death of 42% and a 32% reduction in any diabetes-related end points compared with the diet-alone group. These results suggest that metformin may provide benefits that drugs that increase insulin levels do not. Other agents, such as acarbose and the thiazolidinediones, have not been evaluated in controlled clinical trials that examine their impact on microvascular and macrovascular disease.

Thus although reduction in overall CV events with glycemic control have not been dramatic, there is still good reason to lower blood glucose levels in diabetic patients. Reduction of microvascular events does occur and this will also help to correct some of the metabolic abnormalities of the diabetic metabolic syndrome. As emphasized, management of BP and lipid abnormalities is also of great importance.

SELECTED READING

American Diabetes Association. Standards of medical care in diabetes. *Diabetes Care*. 2004;27(suppl 1):S15-S35.

American Diabetes Association. Physical activity/exercise and diabetes. *Diabetes Care*. 2004;27(suppl 1):S58-S62.

Bolli GB, DiMarcho, Park GD, Pramming S, Koivisto VA. Insulin analogues and their potential in the management of diabetes mellitus. *Diabetologia*. 1999;42:1151-1167.

Canga N, De Irala J, Vara E, Duaso MJ, Ferrer A, Martinez-Gonzalez MA. Intervention study for smoking cessation in diabetic patients: a randomized controlled trial in both clinical and primary care setting. *Diabetes Care*. 2000;23:1455-1460.

Capes SE, Hunt D, Malmberg K, Gerstein HC. Stress hyperglycemia and increased risk of death after myocardial infarction in patients with and without diabetes: a systematic overview. *Lancet*. 2000;355:773-778.

Davidson MB, Peters AL. An overview of metformin in the treatment of type 2 diabetes mellitus. *Am J Med*. 1997;102:99-110.

Jacober SJ, Sowers JR. An update on perioperative management of diabetes. *Arch Intern Med*. 1999;159:2405-2411.

Mahler RJ, Adler ML. Clinical review 102: type 2 diabetes mellitus: update on diagnosis, pathophysiology, and treatment. *J Clin Endocrinol Metab*. 1999;84:1165-1170.

McFarlane SI, Banerji M, Sowers JR. Insulin resistance and cardiovascular disease. *J Clin Endocrinol Metab*. 2001;86:713-718.

UK Prospective Diabetes Study Group. Intensive blood-glucose control with sulphonylureas or insulin compared with conventional treatment and risk of complications in patients with type 2 diabetes (UKPDS 33). *Lancet*. 1998;352:837-853.

The Diabetes Control and Complications Trial Research Group. The effect of intensive treatment of diabetes on the development and progression of long-term complications in insulin-dependent diabetes mellitus. *N Engl J Med.* 1993;329:977-986.

Williamson DF. Weight loss and mortality in persons with type 2 diabetes mellitus: a review of the epidemiological evidence. *Exp Clin Endocrinol Diabetes.* 1998;106(suppl 2):14-21.

Williamson DF, Thompson TJ, Thun M, Flanders D, Pamuk E, Byers T. Intentional weight loss mortality among overweight individuals with diabetes. *Diabetes Care.* 2000;23:1499-1504.

11 Risk Reduction in Special Populations

Treatment Considerations in Women

■ Background

Women are more susceptible to cardiovascular disease (CVD) following menopause for a number of reasons. Low-density lipoprotein (LDL) cholesterol levels are often lower in premenopausal women than those in men, rising to higher levels after menopause than in men. Triglyceride and lipoprotein (a) (LP[a]) levels rise and high-density lipoprotein (HDL) levels fall after menopause. Low HDL cholesterol is a strong predictor of coronary heart disease (CHD) in women and, in the Lipids Research Clinics Follow-up Study, was second only to age as a predictor of CVD death. Trials of statins in secondary prevention of CVD, such as the Scandinavian Simvastatin Survival Study (4S) and Cholesterol and Recurrent Events (CARE), indicate that women benefit similarly to men. The CARE trial even suggests that they may benefit more as a result of their higher absolute risk if they have had a myocardial infarction (MI) or stroke.

■ Diabetes in Women

Diabetes eliminates most of the protection normally afforded by female sex hormones in premenopausal women. Mortality rates from CHD are between three and seven times higher in diabetic women compared with nondiabetic women in contrast to the 2-fold to 4-fold increase in diabetic vs nondiabetic men.

CVD is the leading cause of death in women in the United States, accounting for 30% of all deaths.

Over 235,000 women die annually from acute MI, and >88,000 women die from stroke. The incidence of CHD increases with age, and women >75 years of age constitute the most rapidly growing segment of our population. The mortality from CVD is worse in women than in men, as women typically have more risk factors (ie, systolic hypertension and glucose intolerance) than do men presenting with their initial MI or stroke. Thus the increase in CVD in women parallels the increasing incidence of both diabetes and hypertension.

Increasing obesity in adult women increases the risk for both diabetes and hypertension. Questionnaire data from the Nurses' Health Study cohort of 114,824 women reported that the risk for diabetes increased considerably when the body mass index was >22 kg/m^2. Weight gain after the age of 18 years was strongly related to the risk for developing type 2 diabetes. In contrast, women who lost >5 kg from early adult life had a significantly reduced risk for development of diabetes. These data suggest that any weight gain in women during adulthood increases their risk of developing type 2 diabetes.

Women with diabetes are also more likely to die after an MI than women who do not have diabetes or men with or without diabetes. The risk of death from CHD in women with diabetes is more than three times that in nondiabetic women. As in men, an MI may be "silent" in diabetic women, ie, infarctions (even fatal ones) can occur with little or no chest pain only to be discovered at autopsy or in a routine echocardiogram. Many risk factors contribute to the increase in CVD in diabetic women, including endothelial dysfunction, hypercoagulability, abnormalities of platelet function, dyslipidemia, and hypertension. Thus as for diabetic men, women with this disease should be treated with aspirin, have their LDL cholesterol lowered to <100 mg/dL, and their blood pressure (BP) treated to a goal of <130/80-85 mm Hg.

■ Role of Hormone Replacement Therapy in Diabetic Women

Recent data have questioned whether diabetic postmenopausal women should receive hormone replacement therapy (HRT). There had been circumstantial evidence from the Postmenopausal Estrogen/Progestin Interventions (PEPI) trial that HRT would improve lipids in women who are not diabetic and who have not had prior CVD events. In a case-control study of 334 diabetic women, the use of postmenopausal estrogen replacement was not associated with an increased risk of CVD. However, there are reasons for concern about starting HRT in diabetic women. First, the risk of endometrial carcinoma is increased in diabetic women. Second, as noted repeatedly, persons who have diabetes but who do not have evidence of vascular disease manifest the same risk for MI and stroke as nondiabetic persons who have already had such events. Accordingly, it would be anticipated that diabetic women would respond to HRT similarly to women with CVD, ie, as in the Heart and Estrogen/Progestin Replacement Study (HERS) where the risk of a CHD event was increased in women who received HRT.

Treatment Considerations in Patients With Renal Disease

Control of both glycemia and BP is important in slowing the progression of renal disease in patients with either type 1 or type 2 diabetes. Systolic hypertension is a powerful promotor of renal disease progression in such patients. The rate of decline of renal function in patients with diabetic nephropathy is a continuous function of systolic BP levels down to approximately 125 mm Hg and diastolic BP levels down to 70 to 75 mm Hg. One observational study showed that patients whose systolic BP was maintained <140 mm Hg did not display any deterioration in renal function. Conversely, those with systolic BP levels >140 mm Hg showed a substantial decline in renal function.

In a prospective interventional study of type 1 diabetic patients with hypertension, lowering mean arterial pressure from 143/96 to 130/84 mm Hg with β-blockers and diuretics slowed the decline in glomerular filtration rate by 77%. The Collaborative Study Group showed a 51% slower time to dialysis and doubling of serum creatinine among type 1 hypertensive diabetic patients who received an angiotensin-converting enzyme (ACE) inhibitor in addition to other agents compared with a regimen that did not include an ACE inhibitor. Further, these differences could not be completely explained by significant differences in arterial BP. This advantage of ACE inhibitors in protecting renal function in diabetic patients has been confirmed in longer-term studies in both type 1 and type 2 diabetic patients. Patients with severe renal disease and a nephrotic syndrome also appear to benefit from ACE therapy. Finally, it is clear from a number of long-term studies that those persons with diabetes who achieve BP levels of ≤130/80 mm Hg have the slowest rates of decline in renal function. In a retrospective analysis of the Modified Dietary Protein in Renal Disease (MDRD) trial, those who had >1 g/day of proteinuria, regardless of etiology, had slower rates of renal disease progression when the BP was <125/75 mm Hg. The results of the recent African American Study of Kidney Disease (AASK) also suggest that the use of an ACE inhibitor–based program is beneficial in reducing overall morbidity and mortality in patients with nephropathy, especially in those with significant proteinuria. However, in this study, patients who achieved BP levels <130/80 mm Hg did not experience a better outcome than those with less rigid BP control.

The results of Reduction of Endpoints in Non-insulin Dependent Diabetes Mellitus With an Angiotensin II Antagonist, Losartan (RENAAL), Irbesartan Diabetic Nephropathy Trial (IDNT), and Irbesartan Microalbuminuria Type 2 Diabetes Mellitus in Hypertensive Patients Trial (IRMA 2) indicate that a regimen that includes the use of an angiotensin II receptor blocker (ARB) in type 2 diabetic patients with evidence of renal disease will slow the progression of renal disease and reduce proteinuria to a significant degree compared with regimens that do not include an ARB.

Thus all diabetic patients with microalbuminuria should be receiving an ACE inhibitor or an ARB and should have their BP controlled to <130/80-85 mm Hg. This usually will require multiple medications, one of which should be a diuretic. At present, if significant proteinuria (ie, ≥1 g) is present, BP should be treated to an even more rigorous goal (ie, 125/75 mm Hg), if at all possible.

SELECTED READINGS

Abu-Hamden DR, Sowers JR. Diabetes, dyslipidemia and renal disease in the elderly. *CVR&R*. 1998;2:60-64.

Bakris GL, Williams M, Dworkin L, et al for the National Kidney Foundation Hypertension and Diabetes Executive Committees Working Group. Preserving renal function in adults with hypertension and diabetes: a consensus approach. *Am J Kidney Dis*. 2000;36:645-661.

Kanaya AM, Grady D, Barrett-Connor E. Explaining the sex difference in coronary heart disease mortality among patients with type 2 diabetes: a meta-analysis. *Arch Intern Med*. 2002;162:1737-1745.

Kaseta JB, Skafar DF, Ram JL, Jacober SJ, Sowers JR. Cardiovascular disease in the diabetic woman. *J Clin Endocrinol Metab*. 1999;84:1835-1838.

Natarajan S, Liao Y, Cao G, Lipsitz SR, McGee DL. Sex differences in risk for coronary heart disease mortality associated with diabetes and established coronary heart disease. *Arch Intern Med*. 2003;163:1735-1740.

Sowers JR. Diabetes and cardiovascular disease in women. *Arch Intern Med*. 1998;158:617-621.

12 Target Organs and Diabetes

Stroke in Diabetic Patients

Stroke is the third leading cause of death in the United States. There are >700,000 strokes annually and >4.5 million stroke survivors. Recent epidemiologic data indicate that there has been a recent leveling off of stroke-related mortality but possibly an increase in stroke incidence. It has been suggested that high-risk or stroke-prone persons should be targeted for aggressive, preventive measures and specific interventions. Diabetes is an important and independent modifiable stroke-risk factor of increasing significance as the prevalence of diabetes increases, our population ages, and mortality from other causes decreases.

The worldwide incidence of stroke among patients with diabetes is more than three times that in the general population, with especially high risks in Scandinavian countries and the southeastern United States. Among Hawaiian Japanese men in the Honolulu Heart Program, the diabetic patients had twice the risk of thromboembolic stroke as nondiabetics, independent of other factors known to predispose to stroke. In the Framingham Heart Study, people with glucose intolerance had double the risk for stroke compared with nondiabetics; the relative risk was greater in diabetic women compared with men, especially in the group 40 to 60 years of age.

Patients presenting with stroke are more likely to have undiagnosed type 2 diabetes as well as serum glucose levels >120 mg/dL at 1 hour after a 50-g glucose load. Proteinuria is also a risk factor for stroke, both in people with impaired glucose tolerance and diabetes. African Americans and Caribbean Hispanics have a >2-fold increased incidence of stroke compared with white patients, perhaps reflecting the greater propensity for both diabetes and hypertension in these ethnic groups.

Both short-term and long-term mortality are increased in diabetic patients experiencing a stroke. The increased mortality following a stroke parallels glucose levels. Higher glucose levels also have an unfavorable prognostic value for morbidity.

Hypertension is common in diabetic patients. In an 8-year observation of patients in the United Kingdom Prospective Diabetes Study (UKPDS), the increased risk of stroke in diabetic persons was strongly associated with the degree of blood pressure (BP) elevation, particularly systolic BP (SBP) elevation. Even diabetic patients with SBP between 125 and 142 mm Hg had twice as high a risk for stroke as persons with lower SBP.

■ Stroke Prevention in Diabetic Patients

As noted, data from the UKPDS also showed a 44% relative risk reduction for stroke in the group whose BP was controlled (mean BP of 144/82 mm Hg) compared with the groups with poorer BP control (mean BP of 154 mm Hg). This 44% risk reduction was even greater than the 20% observed in diabetic patients in the Systolic Hypertension in the Elderly Program (SHEP). Tight control of BP was a more significant factor in lowering risk of any diabetes-related end point than intensive blood glucose control.

The nitrendipine-based antihypertensive therapy trial (Systolic Hypertension in Europe [Syst-Eur] multicenter trial) also demonstrated that an excess risk of stroke associated with diabetes was abolished by rigorous antihypertensive treatment of older patients with type 2 diabetes and isolated systolic hypertension. In diabetic patients in the Micro-Hope subanalysis of the Heart Outcomes Prevention Evaluation (HOPE) study, there was a reduction of stroke by 33% with angiotensin-converting enzyme (ACE) inhibitor therapy superimposed on other antihypertensive drugs, antiplatelet therapy (primarily aspirin), lipid-lowering therapy (primarily 3-hydroxy-3-methylglytaryl coenzyme A [HMG-CoA] reductase inhibitor therapy), anticoagulants, and nitrates compared with therapy that did not include an ACE inhibitor.

The benefits of diuretic therapy as part of a regimen designed to reduce BP, especially SBP, were clearly established for the relatively large diabetic cohort in the Antihypertensive and Lipid-Lowering Treatment to Prevent Heart Attack Trial (ALLHAT). Other studies have demonstrated the beneficial effects of angiotensin II receptor blockers (ARBs) and diuretic/ACE inhibitor combinations in the primary and secondary preventions, respectively, of stroke in diabetic patients.

■ Atrial Fibrillation/Anticoagulation

The observational data from the UKPDS also identified atrial fibrillation as an important risk factor for stroke in diabetic patients; diabetic patients between 35 and 74 years of age who had atrial fibrillation on an electrocardiogram (ECG) were eight times more likely to suffer a stroke during the first 8 years of the study than those who were in sinus rhythm. In an 8-year population-based study of persons aged 35 to 74 years, 15.1% of diabetic patients with stroke had previously documented atrial fibrillation compared with 10.7% of those without diabetes.

Warfarin therapy has been shown to be associated with a two-thirds reduction in the risk of stroke when given for atrial fibrillation. The role of anticoagulants in the secondary prevention of stroke in patients with atrial fibrillation, especially in those with diabetes whose risk of cerebral hemorrhage appears to be less than those without diabetes, is of proven benefit. For primary prevention of stroke, patients with diabetes and atrial fibrillation should be on slightly reduced doses of warfarin in the absence of clear contraindications to maintain an international normalized ratio (INR) range of 2.0 to 3.0. If there are contraindications for warfarin, these patients should be maintained on aspirin therapy (81-325 mg/day).

■ Dyslipidemia

A number of prospective studies have shown a significant reduction in the risk for stroke with the use of lipid-lowering drugs in patients with increased risk for thromboembolic stroke, including people with diabetes. These studies include the Scandinavian Simvastatin Survival Study (4S), the Cholesterol and Recurrent Events (CARE) trial, the Medical Research Council/British Heart Foundation (MRC/BHF) Heart Protection Study, and the Anglo Scandinavian Cardiac Outcome Trial (ASCOT). Recent recommendations from the American Diabetes Association, as well as other agencies, note that statins are indicated in diabetics to achieve a goal low-density lipoprotein (LDL) of <100 mg/dL for the primary prevention of stroke as well as myocardial infarction (MI). Careful attention to reducing BP, lipid levels, and glucose levels in diabetic populations will be helpful in reducing the occurrence of carotid artery lesions, a frequent precursor of stroke.

■ Summary

In conclusion, the incidence and severity of stroke are increased in the diabetic patient. Stroke prevention, whether primary or secondary, has proven effective. Prevention measures include rigorous treatment of hypertension, antiplatelet and anticoagulant therapy, and the use of statin therapy. Lifestyle interventions include reduction of dietary salt and fat, smoking cessation, weight reduction, and limitation of alcohol consumption to no more than two drinks per day.

Heart Failure in Diabetes

There is an increased incidence of congestive heart failure (CHF) in diabetes irrespective of coronary artery or hypertensive disease. This unique diabetic cardiac muscle disease is characterized by delayed diastolic relaxation, resulting from a direct effect of hyperglycemia, and altered insulin action on cardiac myocytes, a condition known as diabetic cardiomyopathy. Thus patients with type 2 diabetes have a high incidence of heart failure not only related to increased coronary heart disease and increased hypertensive disease, but also due to diabetic cardiomyopathy.

Framingham Heart Study data revealed a 4-fold greater incidence of CHF in diabetic men and an 8-fold increase in diabetic women compared with nondiabetic persons. Data from the Diabetes Mellitus Insulin-Glucose Infusion in Acute Myocardial Infarction (DIGAMI) trial indicate that CHF accounted for up to 66% of mortality among diabetic patients post-MI during the first year of follow-up. The high incidence of mortality following MI in diabetes is due, in part, to a higher incidence of post-MI CHF as well as arrhythmia-associated death.

Hypertensive cardiomyopathy is a major contributor to CHF in diabetic patients. After adjustment for age and weight, the relationship between increased hypertension and CHF remains.

Hyperglycemia contributes to CHF incidence in patients with diabetes, in part because of increased ischemic cardiomyopathy. The risk of cardiovascular disease (CVD) events, including CHF, rises >1% for every 1% increase in glycosylated hemoglobin A_{1C} (HbA_{1C}). Several trials have shown a trend in reduction of CVD events in diabetic patients with improved glycemic control. Dyslipidemia also contributes to ischemic cardiomyopathy and CVD, as previously discussed.

There is mounting evidence that diabetic cardiomyopathy is related in part to increased angiotensin II overexpression in diabetic hearts, and angiotensin II receptors (AT_1) are significantly up-regulated in diabetic cardiomyocytes. Overexpression of the AT_1 receptor and elevated angiotensin II contributes to both increased fibrosis and apoptosis in diabetic hearts. Both elevated glucose and aldosterone have been shown to stimulate fibrosis and likely contribute significantly to development of CHF in diabetes. Blockade of the renin-angiotensin-aldosterone system (RAAS) with an ACE inhibitor, an ARB, an α-blocker/β-blocker, or a β-blocker may offer a physiologically appropriate approach to preventing and treating CHF in diabetic patients.

Sudden Cardiac Death and Diabetes

Diabetes is associated with a substantial increase in the incidence of sudden cardiac death. The proposed mechanisms for sudden death in diabetic patients include abnormalities of the autonomic nervous system. These abnormalities include enhanced sympathetic activity and diminished parasympathetic activity. ECG abnormalities predisposing to fatal ventricular arrhythmias, such as QTc prolongation and increased QTc dispersion, are found with increased frequency in both type 1 and type 2 diabetes mellitus. Holter monitoring in diabetic patients has shown that the diurnal and nocturnal levels of low frequency/high frequency heart rates, an index of parasympathetic to sympathetic balance, is significantly reduced in persons with diabetic autonomic neuropathy. The normal day-to-night modulation of QT/RR relation is often altered, with a reversed day-night pattern and an increased nocturnal QT rate dependence. Many individuals with the cardiometabolic syndrome and type 2 diabetes demonstrate reduced RR variability indicative of altered autonomic control. Indeed, persons with the cardiometabolic syndrome are at increased risk for sudden death, up to two to three times more frequent, than in those with normal glucose metabolism. Correction of glycemia, hypertension, and lipid levels, as well as maintaining adequate levels of potassium, magnesium, and chromium intake, may be helpful in reducing the occurrence of sudden death in this population.

■ Current Control of CVD Risk Factors in Diabetic Patients

In a recent retrospective chart-review analysis, only 25% to 30% of diabetic patients were treated to goal BP levels of 130/80 mm Hg. Inadequate treatment largely reflected lack of SBP control. Only 25% to 30% of surveyed patients had achieved HbA_{1C} <7% and 50% still had HbA_{1C} >8%. In another analysis, 35% of diabetic subjects had levels of LDL cholesterol <100 mg/dL but one third had LDL cholesterol levels >130 mg/dL. Data indicate that only 50% of eligible diabetic patients are treated with aspirin. Despite the particularly high risk of CVD among women with diabetes, they are not treated aggressively with lipid therapy and fewer are currently receiving aspirin than men.

SUGGESTED READING

Davis TM, Millns H, Stratton IM, Holman RR, Turner RC. Risk factors for stroke in type 2 diabetes mellitus: United Kingdom Prospective Diabetes Study (UKPDS) 29. *Arch Intern Med*. 1999;159:1097-1103.

Effects of ramipril on cardiovascular and microvascular outcomes in people with diabetes mellitus: results of the HOPE study and MICRO-HOPE substudy. Heart Outcomes Prevention Evaluation Study Investigators. *Lancet*. 2000;355:253-259.

Fagan TC, Sowers J. Type 2 diabetes mellitus: greater cardiovascular risks and greater benefits of therapy. *Arch Intern Med*. 1999;159:1033-1034.

Gustafsson I, Hildebrandt P. Early failure of the diabetic heart. *Diabetes Care*. 2001;24:3-4.

Haffner SM. Coronary heart disease in patients with diabetes. *N Engl J Med*. 2000;342:1040-1042.

Lindholm LH, Ibsen H, Dahlof B, et al; LIFE Study Group. Cardiovascular morbidity and mortality in patients with diabetes in the Losartan Intervention For Endpoint reduction in hypertension study (LIFE): a randomised trial against atenolol. *Lancet*. 2002;359:1004-1010.

PROGRESS Collaborative Group. Randomised trial of a perindopril-based blood-pressure-lowering regimen among 6,105 individuals with previous stroke or transient ischaemic attack. *Lancet*. 2001;358:1033-1041.

Sacco RL. Reducing the risk of stroke in diabetes: what have we learned that is new? *Diabetes Obes Metab*. 2002;4(suppl 1):S27-S34.

Sowers JR. Hypertension, angiotensin II, and oxidative stress. *N Engl J Med*. 2002;346:1999-2001

Valensi PE, Johnson NB, Maison-Blanche P, Extramania F, Motte G, Coumel P. Influence of cardiac autonomic neuropathy on heart rate dependence of ventricular repolarization in diabetic patients. *Diabetes Care*. 2002;25:918-923.

13 Summary of Cardiovascular Disease Reduction in Diabetics

Cardiovascular disease (CVD) accounts for up to 80% of mortal events in persons with diabetes. Thus all strategies to reduce this risk should be optimized in these patients. All patients who tolerate aspirin should receive a minimum aspirin dose of 81 mg/day up to one adult aspirin 325 mg/day. Further, since diabetic patients without evidence of vascular disease have the same CVD risk as nondiabetics who have already had a myocardial infarction (MI) or stroke, their low-density lipoprotein (LDL) cholesterol should be lowered at least to <100 mg/dL or, if at all possible, to <70 mg/dL. Importantly, blood pressure (BP) should be lowered, if necessary, and maintained at as close as possible to optimal levels of about 120/80 mm Hg. If they can tolerate an angiotensin-converting enzyme (ACE) inhibitor, they should receive one of these agents (usually in addition to a low-dose diuretic). A β-blocker or angiotensin II receptor blocker (ARB) (usually with a low-dose diuretic) are also appropriate therapies. The addition of a calcium antagonist may be necessary to lower BP to <130/80-85 mm Hg. Data from ongoing studies suggest that the use of an ARB may prove to be interchangeable with an ACE inhibitor in therapy without concerns for a cough.

Optimal glycemic control should be attempted, even though this strategy has not been proven consistently to lower CVD risk. It is critical to engage diabetic patients in hygienic measures, including weight reduction, moderate exercise, discontinuation of smoking, and moderation of alcohol intake. A comprehensive guide to primary prevention of CVD in diabetics is presented in **Table 13.1**.

Summary

The management of diabetes has evolved significantly since the discovery of insulin and the realization that correcting blood glucose abnormalities could slow down or prevent progression of kidney disease, retinopathy, and CVD. During the past 50 years, widespread efforts have been made to regulate blood glucose levels. These initially involved the manipulation of insulin dosage and nutritional interventions. Regimens were complicated, diets were difficult to follow, and insulin reactions were common.

With the discovery that diabetes is part of a complex metabolic syndrome and that insulin resistance plays a major role in the eventual development of diabetes in a majority of patients, a new approach was undertaken. New oral hypoglycemic drugs were marketed. Some of these increased the secretion of insulin; others helped to increase insulin utilization. With the introduction of more effective therapies and less dependence on rigid diets that required careful selections of components of various food groups, management improved. Longevity, both in the insulin-dependent type 1 diabetic and the much more common type 2 diabetic, increased significantly.

In recent years, it has become evident that most of the morbidity/mortality in diabetics is not related to diabetic microvascular events (ie, retinopathy and nephropathy). Although emphasis should still be placed on the prevention of these serious complications, the new paradigm suggests strongly that in the diabetic patient more attention must be placed on the prevention or management of other risk factors. Glycemic control is important, but control of elevated BP, lipid abnormalities, and smoking habits may be more important.

In the *Management of Cardiovascular Risk Factors in Diabetes*, a review and update not only of the lifestyle management components of the diabetic patient, but of other risk factors that may play an even more important role in the outcome of these patients, is presented. Until recent years, little attention has been paid to these important factors:

- A majority of patients with diabetes and hypertension remain untreated and certainly have not reached goal BP levels <130/80-85 mm Hg.
- A majority of diabetic patients, who should be considered as high-risk individuals for CVD and in the same category as nondiabetics who have already experienced a cardiovascular (CV) episode, have not been treated adequately with regard to the management of lipid disorders.
- A majority of hypertensive diabetic patients who have clotting abnormalities are not being treated with simple antiplatelet medications, such as aspirin.

It is important that the management of the diabetic patient be extended beyond nutritional intervention and glycemic control. Diets should be advised and monitored, exercise should be encouraged, weight loss (if appropriate) should be undertaken, and hypoglycemic medications given to control blood glucose levels. Most importantly, as consistently emphasized, BP should be lowered to goal levels that are even lower than in nondiabetics and LDL cholesterol lowered to <70 mg/dL if at all possible, a level that heretofore has been reserved for patients with known coronary heart disease. In addition, efforts should be made to decrease triglyceride levels to <150 mg/dL, and to raise HDL levels to > 45 mg/dL if they are low.

TABLE 13.1 — Guide to Prevention of Cardiovascular Disease in Patients With Diabetes*

Risk Intervention	Goal(s)	Recommendations	
BP control	<130/80-85 mm Hg	Measure BP at each visit; consider home BP monitoring. Promote lifestyle modification: weight control, physical activity, moderation in alcohol, moderate sodium restriction. Antihypertensive medication usually necessary: begin medical therapy if BP >130/85 mm Hg along with lifestyle modifications (JNC 7 suggests use of medication in addition to lifestyle changes as soon as diagnosis is made); two medications as initial therapy may be appropriate	
Cholesterol management		Ask about dietary habits as part of routine evaluation. Measure total and HDL cholesterol and TG; estimate LDL	
	Primary goal: LDL at least <100 mg/dL and to <70 mg/dL, if possible; Rule out secondary causes of high LDL (liver or thyroid abnormalities)	Start diet (<25% total fat; <7% saturated fat, <200 mg/dL cholesterol) and weight control. Consider adding drug therapy to diet therapy for LDL levels >100 mg/dL	Other risk factors that may increase the importance of lipid control include hypertension, smoking history, and family history of CHD in male relatives <55 Y/A and in female relatives <65 Y/A

	Secondary goal: HDL >35 mg/dL; TG <200 mg/dL	Suggested drug therapy for LDL levels >130 mg/dL (drug selection priority modified according to TG level)			
		TG Levels (mg/dL)			HDL <35 mg/dL: emphasize weight management and physical activity, avoidance of cigarette smoking. Consider drug therapy—niacin, which must be used with care in diabetics, or fibrate.
		<200	200–400	>400	
		Statin resin	Statin ± fibrate	Consider combined drug therapy (statin + fibrate)	
		If LDL goal of <100 mg/dL not achieved, consider combination drug therapy (statin + fibrate). Niacin is extremely effective, but must be used with care in diabetics			
Glucose control	Near normal fasting glucose; HbA$_{1C}$ ≤1% above normal (<6.5%)	*First-step therapy:* weight reduction and exercise. *Second-step therapy:* oral hypoglycemic agents (sulfonylureas and/or metformin; ancillary; acarbose, glitazone. *Third-step therapy:* combined oral antidiabetic agents ± insulin therapy			

Continued

Risk Intervention	Goal(s)	Recommendations
Smoking	Complete cessation	Ask about smoking status as part of routine evaluation. Reinforce nonsmoking status. Strongly encourage patient and family to stop smoking. Provide counseling, nicotine replacement, and formal cessation programs as appropriate
Antiplatelet agents	—	Aspirin 81-325 mg/d, if not contraindicated, for primary prevention. Manage warfarin to international normalized ratio 2 to 3.5 for post-MI patients and those with atrial fibrillation
Physical acitivity	Increase amount; exercise regularly 3-4 times/wk for 30 min	Ask about physical activity status and exercise habits as part of routine evaluation. Encourage 30 min of moderate-intensity exercise 3-4 times/wk as well as increased physical activity in daily life. Encourage regular exercise to improve conditioning and reduce CV risk. Advise medically supervised programs for those with low functional capacity and/or comorbidities
Weight management	Achieve and maintain desirable BMI and waist circumference	Measure patient's weight and height, BMI, and waist circumference at each visit as part of routine evaluation. Desirable BMI <25 kg/m^2. Desirable waist circumference for men (<38-40 in) and women (<32-34 in)

Estrogens	—	Efficacy for CVD risk reduction in diabetic women not proved. Some evidence in older women of an increase in CVD.
ACE inhibitors (ARBs may be substituted) in post-MI patients	—	Start early post-MI in stable high-risk patients. Continue indefinitely for all with LV dysfunction (EF ≤40%) or symptoms of HF. Use as needed to manage BP
β-Blockers	—	Start in post-MI patients; continue indefinitely. Observe usual contraindications. Appropriate use of β-blockers not contraindicated in diabetic patients. Use as needed to manage angina, rhythm abnormalities, or BP in all other patients

Abbreviations: ACE, angiotensin-converting enzyme; BMI, body mass index; BP, blood pressure; CHD, coronary heart disease; CV, cardiovascular; CVD, cardiovascular disease; EF, ejection fraction; HbA$_{1C}$, glycosylated hemoglobin; HDL, high-density lipoprotein; LDL, low-density lipoprotein; LV, left ventricle; MI, myocardial infarction; TG, triglyceride; Y/A, years of age.

* These patients, without clinical evidence of CVD, are to be considered in the same risk category as nondiabetic patients with CVD (ie, they are high-risk subjects).

The future of patients with type 2 diabetes, patients who now number more than 15 million in the United States, has been dramatically improved. This has occurred by paying more attention to CV risk factors in addition to blood sugar abnormalities. Much more can be done to prolong the lives of diabetics and importantly to decrease mortality from renal as well as CV complications.

Management of Cardiovascular Risk Factors in Diabetes has tried to outline the reasons for a multifaceted approach to the treatment of diabetes. The evolution of the management of diabetes has followed that of the treatment of hypertension. Initially, only symptomatic or severe type 1 diabetics were treated. Malignant hypertension was treated first and, as data were collected from the clinical trials, less severe hypertension was treated. Today, lowering BP in people with stage I disease (140-160/90-100 mm Hg) even without evidence of renal or cardiac disease is justified based on results of randomized clinical trials. Similarly, there are now enough studies in diabetic patients to justify a more aggressive approach to managing CV risk factors in this population, even in those without evidence of CVD.

As noted elsewhere in this book, management need not be complicated, expensive, or involved. Complicated procedures or frequent doctor visits may not be necessary. Most patients can modify their lifestyle and adhere to therapy for lowering BP and correct at least most of the lipid abnormalities as well as their blood glucose levels without turning their households into diet kitchens or radically changing their life.

SELECTED READING

Moser M, Ross H. The treatment of hypertension in diabetic patients. *Diabetes Care*. 1993;16:542-547.

Sowers JR. Treatment of hypertension in patients with diabetes. *Arch Intern Med*. 2004;164:1850-1857.

INDEX

Note: Page numbers in *italics* indicate figures;
page numbers followed by t refer to tables.

A-V nicking, 172
AASK, 152, 238-239
ABCD trial. See *Appropriate Blood Pressure Control in Diabetes.*
Abdominal obesity
  age-related, 42, 46
  exercise and, after menopause, 46
  hypertension and, 26t
  insulin resistance and, 26t, 45
  metabolic and cardiovascular risk factors and, 25, 26t
  in metabolic syndrome, 40t
  microalbuminuria and, 62t
Acarbose (Precose)
  action mechanism of, 229
  dosage of, 223t-224t
  indications for, 253t
  metformin with, 225
  side effects of, 229
  type 2 diabetes development and, 26
  vascular disease and, 232
Accupril (quinapril), *140,* 154t
ACE inhibitors. See *Angiotensin-converting enzyme inhibitors.*
Acebutolol (Sectral), 165t
Aceon (perindopril), 154t
Actos. See *Pioglitazone.*
ADA. See *American Diabetes Association recommendations.*
Adhesion molecules, ACE inhibitors and, 79
Adolescents, diabetes type 2 diagnosis in, 26
Advicor (niacin/lovastatin), 184t
Aerobic exercise, 143, 213
AFCAPS/TexCAPS, 187, 196
African American Study of Kidney Disease (AASK), 152, 238-239
Age
  at diabetes onset, 18
  hypertension and, in diabetes, 39
  at hypertension onset, 47-48
Aging
  abdominal obesity and, 42, 46
  cardiovascular disease and, 37-39
  diabetes and
    prevalence of, 19, *20-22*
    testing for, 27t
  hypertension and, 42, 47-48
  and progression from impaired glucose tolerance to diabetes, 24
  skeletal muscle loss in, 42
Air Force/Texas Coronary Atherosclerosis Prevention Study
  (AFCAPS/TexCAPS), 187, 196
Albuminuria
  ACE inhibitors and, 101
  ADA recommendations on, 142
  definition of, 36t
  management of, 172-173
  progressive increase in, 67
Alcohol intake, 143, 143t, 145t, 212t, 249, 252t
Aldactazide (spironolactone/hydrochlorothiazide), 170t
Aldoril (methyldopa/hydrochlorothiazide), 170t
Aldosterone. See also *Renin-angiotensin-aldosterone system.*
  ACE inhibitors and ARB actions on, *74,* 89, 157t

257

Aldosterone *(continued)*
  congestive heart failure and, in diabetes, 246
  in hypertension pathogenesis, *50*
  production and functions of, 73, 75
ALLHAT. See *Antihypertensive and Lipid-Lowering Treatment to Prevent Heart Attack Trial.*
α-Blockers, 87. See also specific drugs.
  β-Blockers with, for hypertension, 165t
  in congestive heart failure, 246
α-Glucosidase inhibitors. See also specific drugs.
  action mechanisms of, 229
  adverse effects of, 229
  dosage of, 223t
  indications for, *226-227*
α-Methyldopa, 107
Altace. See *Ramipril.*
Altocor. See *Lovastatin.*
Amaryl. See *Glimepiride.*
American Diabetes Association (ADA) recommendations
  on albuminuria, 142
  on aspirin therapy, 203-204
  on blood pressure goals, 120, 150
  on diagnostic criteria for diabetes, 28t
  dietary, 193, 213
  on glycemic control, 209t
  on initial hypertension therapies, 155, 194
  on statins, 244
American Heart Association (AHA) dietary recommendations, 193
Amiloride/hydrochlorothiazide (Moduretic), 170t
Amlodipine
  ACE inhibitor with, 173
  dosage of, 125, 156, 169t, 171
  effectiveness of, 104-105, 156
  fosinopril vs, in FACET. See *Fosinopril vs Amlodipine Cardiovascular Event Trial (FACET).*
  renal disease and, *124,* 125, *126*
  with/without fosinopril, cardiovascular events and, 167, *167*
Amlodipine/benazepril (Lotrel), 169t
Amputation, diabetes-related, 218
ANBP-2, 82t, 86t
Angina
  β-blockers in, 110, 255
  in diabetics vs nondiabetics, 38
  exercise thallium scan and, 172
  on FACET, 85, 106t, 132t
  nitric oxide metabolism in, 56
  unstable, pravastatin for, 181
Angiotensin-converting enzyme (ACE) inhibitors. See also specific drugs.
  action mechanisms of, *51,* 57, 75-78, 104, 154t
  action sites of, *74*
  ARB interchangeability with, 249
  ARBs vs, 153, 156
  β-blocker with/without diuretic vs, 101-102, 109t, 109-110, *114,* 115t
  bradykinin and, *74,* 79
  calcium channel blockers vs, 152
  calcium channel blockers with, 166-167, 169t, 173
  cardiovascular effects of, 79, 88, 110-111, 114, *114,* 129, 131, 131t, 135
  in combination drug therapy, 77, 173
  in diabetic with hypertension, 79, 88-89
  diuretic with, 152, 166, 168t
  dosages of, 154t
  hyperglycemia risk with, *161*
  in hypertensive patient progression to type 2 diabetes, 48-49, *50-51*

258

ACE inhibitors *(continued)*
  indications for, *140*
  insulin resistance and, 76-78, 152-153
  JNC 6 and 7 recommendations on, 114
  for microproteinuria, 70t
  after myocardial infarction, 217t
  proteinuria reduction with, 67-68, 152
  RAAS and, 73, 88-89, 104
  renal disease and, 038-239, 75-76, 101-102, 102t, 104, 131, 131t
    progression of, 66
  side effects of, 154t
  vascular actions of, 79
Angiotensin II. See also *Renin-angiotensin-aldosterone system.*
  in diabetic hearts, 246
  diabetic hypertension and, 55
  insulin resistance and, 48, *50,* 75
  production and functions of, 73, 75
Angiotensin II receptor blockers (ARBs). See also specific drugs.
  ACE inhibitor interchangeability with, 249
  ACE inhibitors vs, 153, 156
  action mechanism of, 49, 88-89, 102, 153, 155, 187t
  action sites of, *74*
  advantages of, 153
  bradykinin and, *74,* 78
  cardiovascular mortality and, 88, 131
  in combination therapy for nephropathy, 102, 123, *124*
  congestive heart failure and, 125
  creatinine clearance and, 125
  in diabetics vs nondiabetics, 129
  diuretics with, 168t-169t
  dosages of, 157t
  hyperglycemia risk with, *161*
  indications for, *140*
  as initial therapy, 155
  losartan vs, 128-129
  microproteinuria and, 70t, 126-127
  proteinuria and, 67-68, 127
  renal disease and, 104, 123-127, 239, *1124*
    progression of, 66
  side effects of, 157t
Anglo Scandinavian Cardiac Outcome Trial (ASCOT), 179, 244
Anticoagulation therapy, in diabetic stroke prevention, 243-244
Antihypertensive and Lipid-Lowering Treatment to Prevent Heart Attack Trial (ALLHAT)
  ACE inhibitors and glucose metabolism on, 81t
  ACE inhibitors vs diuretics and calcium channel blockers on, 86t-87t
  angiotensin and insulin action on, 48
  calcium channel blockers on, 86t-87t, 166
  coronary heart disease events on, 151, 166
  diuretics on, 81t, 86t-87t, 243
  new-onset diabetes on, 82t, 86t
  renal disease progression on, 151, 166
  size and duration of, 82t, 151
Antihypertensive drugs. See also specific drug or drug type.
  adverse effects of
    in diabetics vs nondiabetics, 98, 99t
    glycemic and lipid changes as, 15
  in combination with other drug types, 168t-169t
  stepped-care regimen in, 92-93, 93t
Antiplatelet Trialists Collaboration, 203
Antithrombin III, 58t, 59
Apolipoprotein B concentration, abdominal obesity and, 26t

Appropriate Blood Pressure Control in Diabetes (ABCD)
  ACE inhibitors in, calcium channel blockers vs, 152
  enalapril vs nisoldipine or amlodipine on, 104-106, 105t
  overall results of, 85, 132t
  RAAS inhibitors and calcium channel blockers in, 152
  termination of, 85
ARBs. See *Angiotensin II receptor blockers.*
ASCOT, 179, 244
Aspirin therapy
  action mechanisms of, 204-205
  ADA guidelines for, 203-204
  blood pressure control and, 120
  contraindications for, 204
  in diabetes, 247
  dosage in, 172, 203-205, 244, 249, 254t
  in HOPE study, 243
  in HOT trial, 120, 204
  in hypertension, 47, 251
  indications for, 68, 172, 179, 203-204, 236, 251, 254t
  preventive, 63, 203-204
  in women, 236-237, 247
Atacand. See *Candesartan.*
Atacand HCT (candesartan/hydrochlorothiazide), 168t
Atenolol (Tenormin)
  action mechanisms of, 164t
  with chlorthalidone, 94, 133t
    in SHEP, 94, 100, 133t
  in diabetes, 88, 109t
  dosage of, 94, 107, 164t
  in LIFE study, 128-129, *130*
  losartan vs, 128-129, *130*
  in UKPDS, 85, 88, 107, 109t
  vascular complications and, 158
Atenolol/chlorthalidone (Tenoretic), 169t
Atherosclerosis
  in AFCAPS/TexCAPS, 187
  endothelial dysfunction in, 57-58, 62-63
  glomerulosclerosis and, 61
  lipid abnormalities and, 56, 176-177
  premature, abdominal obesity and, 26t
  proteinuria and, 64-65
  RAAS blockade and, 104
Atorvastatin (Lipitor)
  clinical study of, 179, 187, 198t
  dosage and availability of, 183t, 199t
  effects on lipids, 199t
Atrial fibrillation, in diabetes, 243-244
Australian National Blood Pressure-2 (ANBP-2), 82t, 86t
Autoimmune pancreatic β-cell destruction, 20-21
Autonomic neuropathy, 17
  nondipping and, 53
Avalide (irbesartan/hydrochlorothiazide), *141*, 168t
Avandamet (rosiglitazone/metformin), 224t
Avandia. See *Rosiglitazone.*
Avapro. See *Irbesartan* entries.

Baroreceptor sensitivity, 55
Baroreflex, nondipping and, 53
Bedtime glucose, 209t
Benazepril (Lotensin), 154t
Benazepril/hydrochlorothiazide (Lotensin HCT), 168t
Benazepril with amlodipine (Lotrel), 169t

Bendroflumethiazide
  dosage of, *141*
  with nadolol (Corzide), *141,* 169t
Benicar (olmesartan), 157t, 169t
Beta-blockers. See also *Captopril Prevention Project Study;* specific drugs.
  ACE inhibitors vs, 101-102, 109t, 109-110
  action mechanism of, 164t-165t
  α-blockers with, for hypertension, 165t
  cardiovascular events and, 133t
  chlorthalidone with, in HDFP, 92
  in diabetics, 88
    new-onset, 78, 100-101, 160
    safety of, 88, 100, 110, 150, 160, *161,* 163
  diuretics with, 88, 98-99, 102, *114,* 132t, *140,* 163, 166, 169t
  dosages of, 164t-165t
  effectiveness of, 88, 98-99, 115t, 133t, 163, 164t-165t, 166
  indications for, *140,* 255t
  with intrinsic sympathomimetic action, 165t
  RAAS and, 88
  side effects of, 15
β-Cells
  autoimmune destruction of, 20-21
  dysfunctional, in diabetes type 2 pathogenesis, 30
  insulin secretory response of, 21, 23
Biguanide, 220, 223t
  with sulfonylureas, 224t
  with thiazolidinedione, 224t
Biofeedback, 143t
Birth weight of offspring, diabetes testing and, 27t
Bisoprolol (Zebeta)
  action mechanisms of, 164t
  diuretic with, *141*
  dosage of, 164t
Bisoprolol/hydrochlorothiazide (Ziac), *141,* 169t
Black population
  diabetes in
    prevalence of, 19, 24
    testing for, 27t
  renal disease in, 238
Blindness, diabetic retinopathy and, 28, 217
Blocadren (timolol), 164t
Blood coagulation abnormalities
  abdominal obesity and, 26t
  aspirin therapy for, 251
  cardiovascular disease and, 25, 39
  in diabetes, 13
    examples of, 58t
    mechanism of, 58-60
  hormone replacement therapy and, 38
  microalbuminuria and, 62t
  as risk factor, 25, 39
Blood coagulation disorders, in hypertension, 13, 47
Blood coagulation factors VII and VIII, 58, 58t
Blood flow, in skeletal muscle, in hypertension, 46-47
Blood pressure. See also *Hypertension.*
  ADA recommendations on, 120, 150
  aspirin therapy and, 47, 120, 251
  diastolic
    cardiovascular risk and, 118, *118*
    in HOT trial, 122
    vascular rigidity and, 122
  dippers vs nondippers, 53, *54*

Blood pressure *(continued)*
  goal levels for, 252t
    in diabetics, 93, 139, *140*
    in nondiabetics, 93
  labile, in diabetics, 139
  lowering of, cardiovascular events and, 15
  measurement of
    at home, 141, 173, 252t
    posture during, 142
  National Kidney Foundation recommendations for
    in diabetics, 120, 150
    in nondiabetics, 120
  nighttime
    left ventricular hypertrophy and, 53
    microalbuminuria and, 53
  renal disease and, in diabetes, 237-238
  at same level in diabetics and nondiabetics, cardiovascular disease mortality and, 93-94, 97-98
  systolic
    cardiovascular disease and, 31, 40, *41*, 118, *118*
    coronary heart disease and, 16
    dippers vs nondippers, 53, *53*
    goal for, 16
    macrovascular and microvascular complications and, 16
    microalbuminuria and, 62t, 64
    renal disease progression and, 66
Blood pressure cuff, for obese patients, 139
Body mass index
  calculation of, 146, 147t
  in diabetes type 2 diagnosis, 26
  in women, 236
Bradykinin, *74, 79*

Calcium channel blockers. See also specific drugs.
  ACE inhibitors vs, 152
  ACE inhibitors with, 166-167, 169t
  as add-on vs initial therapy, 163
  cardiovascular effects of, 132t, 135
  enalapril vs, 104-106, 105t
  indications for, *140*, 163, 166, 249
  RAAS inhibitors vs, 152
  renal disease and, *124*, 125-126
  safety of, 15, 106, *161*, 166
  trials of, 163, 166
Calcium intake, 143t
Calories, to maintain or lose weight, 146, 148t, 212t
Candesartan (Atacand)
  action mechanisms of, 157t
  adverse reactions to, 157t
  diuretic in, *141*
  dosage of, *141*, 157t
  enalapril with, 155
Candesartan/hydrochlorothiazide (Atacand HCT), 168t
Capillary endothelium, accelerated disappearance of, 58
Capoten. See *Captopril.*
CAPPP. See *Captopril Prevention Project.*
Captopril (Capoten)
  action mechanism of, 154t
  adverse reactions to, 154t
  diabetic nephropathy and, 103t, 152
  dosage of, 107, 154t
  proteinuria and, 155
  vascular effectiveness of, 158

Captopril/hydrochlorothiazide (Captozide), 168t
Captopril Prevention Project (CAPPP)
  ACE inhibitors in
    β-blockers/diuretics vs, 110-111, *114*
    in combination therapy, 152
    diabetes development and, 76
    new-onset diabetes and, 76
  diabetic hypertensive patients on, 85, 86t, 822t
  insulin resistance and angiotensin II in, 48
  overall results of, 132t
  risk reduction in, 115t
  size and procedures in, 110-111
Captozide (captopril/hydrochlorothiazide), 168t
Carbohydrates
  agents that delay absorption of, 229-230
  dietary, 212t, 1820
Cardiac death, sudden, in diabetes, 246-247
Cardiometabolic syndrome
  insulin resistance in, 29, 51
  progression to type 2 diabetes and cardiovascular events, 51, 63
Cardiovascular disease/events. See also *Coronary heart disease.*
  age and, 37-38
  blood coagulation abnormalities and, 39
  cardiometabolic syndrome progression to, 51, 63
  death from, 14, 37-39
    ACE inhibitors and, 88, 111, *114,* 115t, 129, 132t-133t
    ARBs and, 88, 131
    atenolol vs losartin in, *130*
    in diabetics, reasons for, 63
    in diabetics and nondiabetics at same blood pressure, 94, 98
    diuretics with beta-blockers and, 98-99
    gender and, 33, 235-236
    microalbuminuria and, *69*
    pravastatin and, 181, 185, *188-189,* 189
    pravastatin in, 181, 185, 187, *188-189*
    prevalence of, 33
    ramipril and, 79
  in diabetic women, 38-39
  endothelial dysfunction and, 39
  estrogen protection from, diabetes and, 38
  family history of, 39, 171
  glucose control and, marginal success of, 13
  hypertension and, 39-42, *41*
  lipoprotein abnormalities and, 25, 39
  menopause and, 38, 235
  obesity and, 39, 42
  platelet aggregation/adhesion and, 39
  risk of, in diabetic vs nondiabetic population, 34, *35*
  systolic vs diastolic blood pressure and, *118,* 118-119
  vascular compliance and, 39
  vascular oxidative stress and, 39
CARDS, 179, 198t
CARE study. See *Cholesterol and Recurrent Events study.*
Carvedilol (Coreg), in diabetics, 160-161, 162t, 163
Casual (nonfasting) plasma glucose, 27
Cavus feet, 219t
Central antiadrenergic agents, hyperglycemia risk with, *161*
Cerebrovascular disease. See *Stroke.*
Charcot's joint, 219t
CHARM, 82t, 87t
Chest pain, exercise and, 215
Children, diabetes type 2 diagnosis in, 26

Chlorthalidone (Hygroton, Thalitone), 159t
  atenolol with, 94, 100, 133t
  clonidine with (Clorpres), 170t
  dosage of, 159t
    in HDFP, 92
    in SHEP, 94
  drugs added to, 94
  reserpine with (Diupres), 170t
  safety of, 158
Cholesterol and Recurrent Events (CARE) study
  cardiovascular disease in women on, 235
  coronary artery death on, 186t
  coronary heart disease on, 181
  dyslipidemia and stroke on, 244
  nonfatal myocardial infarction on, 186t
  pravastatin on, 198t
  size of, 185, 186t, 200t
  statins and diabetes on, 181, 185, 187, 196
Cholesterol intake, 178t, 212t, 252t
  in dyslipidemia treatment, 178t
Cholesterol management, 252t-253t
Cholestyramine (Questran, Questran Light, Prevalite), 182t
Clonidine/chlorthalidone (Clorpres), 170t
Clopidogrel (Plavix), 205
Clorpres (clonidine/chlorthalidone), 170t
Coagulation abnormalities. See *Blood coagulation abnormalities*.
Coagulation factors VII and VIII, 49, 49t
Colesevelam (WelChol), 182t
Colestid (colestipol), 182t
Colestipol (Colestid), 182t
Collaborative Atorvastatin Diabetes Study (CARDS), 179, 198t
Collaborative Study Group, ACE inhibitors and renal function findings of, 238
Collagen synthesis, in hyperglycemia, 58
Congestive heart failure
  aldosterone and, 246
  ARBs and, 125
  death from, 33
  in diabetes, 245-246
  simvastatin and, *190*
Coreg (carvedilol), in diabetics, 160-161, 162t, 163
Corgard (nadolol)
  action mechanisms of, 164t
  diuretic with, *141*
  dosage of, 164t
  indications for, *141*
Coronary heart disease. See also *Cardiovascular disease/events*.
  abdominal obesity and, 26t
  on CARE study, 181, 186t
  HDL cholesterol and, 235
  systolic blood pressure and, 16
Corzide (nadolol/bendroflumethiazide), *141*, 169t
Cozaar. See *Losartan*.
Creatinine
  ACE inhibitors and, 102T
  in overnight urine specimen, 67
Creatinine clearance
  ARBs and, 125
  glycemic control and, 68
Crestor (rosuvastatin)
  in diabetics, 180
  dosage of, 183t, 199t
  effect on lipid types, 199t

DAIS. See *Diabetes Atherosclerosis Intervention Study.*
DASH eating plan, 145t, 150
DCCT, 207, 231
Death
  cardiac, sudden, in diabetes, 246-247
  from cardiovascular disease, 14, 33, 37-39
    ACE inhibitors and, 88, 111, *114,* 115t, 129, 132t-133t
    ARBs and, 88, 131
    atenolol vs losartin in, *130*
    in diabetes, reasons for, 63
    in diabetics and nondiabetics at same blood pressure, 94, 98
    diuretics with β-blockers and, 98-99
    gender and, 33, 235-236
    microalbuminuria and, *69*
    pravastatin and, 181, 185, 187, *188-189*
    prevalence of, 33
    ramipril and, 79
  from congestive heart failure, 33
    aldosterone and, 246
    ARBs and, 125
  from myocardial infarction, in women, 38
  from peripheral vascular disease, 33
  from renal disease, 14, 38
  smoking and, diabetes synergism with, 42
  from stroke, 241
  in women, 33, 37-38, *130,* 236
  sudden, 33
Dementia, antihypertensives and, in diabetics vs nondiabetics, 98, 99t
Depression, antihypertensives and, in diabetics vs nondiabetics, 98, 99t
DiaBeta (glyburide), 222t, 231
Diabetes Atherosclerosis Intervention Study (DAIS), 162, 171t
  design of and patient selection for, 191
  dyslipidemia correction and coronary artery disease on, 187, 191, *192*
  fibrates on, 196, 198t
Diabetes Control and Complications Trial (DCCT), 207, 231
Diabetes mellitus
  aging and, 19, *20-22*
  aspirin therapy in, 247
  atenolol in, 88
  β-blocker safety in, 88, 100, 110, 150, 160, *161,* 163
  blood pressure goal in, 91
  clotting disorders in, 13, 59-60
  congestive heart failure in, 245-246
  diagnostic criteria for, 27t-28t, 27-29
    in HDFP, 92-93
  dyslipidemia and, 55-56, 177-178, 178t
  and exclusion from hypertension studies, 91
  exercise precautions in, 214, 215t
  frequency of, 16
  gender and, 19, *22*
  genetics of, 24, 27t
  glycemic goals in, 209t7
  hypertension in. See *Hypertension, in diabetes.*
  life expectancy in, 18-19, *24*
  nephropathy in, 18, 36-37, 76
  neuropathy in, 17, 36, 53
  new-onset
    on ALLHAT, 82t, 86t
    on ANBP-2, 82t
    antihypertensive medications and, 78-79, 82t-83t, 86t-87t, 100-101, 160
    on CAPPP, 76, 82t
    on CHARM, 82t
    on HOPE, 76, 82t, 152-153

Diabetes mellitus, new-onset *(continued)*
  on INSIGHT, 83t
  on INVEST, 83t
  on LIFE, 83t, 87t
  RAAS inhibitors and, 52, 78-79, 101
  on SCOPE, 83t
  on STOP-2, 83t
  on VALUE, 83t156, 151
 obesity incidence in, 13, 19, 146
 onset of, age at, 18
 pravastatin in, in LIPID trial, 181, *188-189*
 progression from impaired glucose tolerance to, 24, 49, *51*
 race/ethnicity and, 19-20, *22*, 24-25, 27t
 simvastatin in, 181
 stroke in
  incidence of, 241-242
  losartan vs atenolol and, *130*
  prevention of, 242-243
 sudden cardiac death and, 246-247
 testing for, 27t
Diabetes Mellitus Insulin-Glucose Infusion in Acute Myocardial Infarction (DIGAMI) trial, 245
Diabetes mellitus type 1, insulin secretion deficiency in, 21
Diabetes mellitus type 2
 cardiometabolic syndrome progression to, 51
 diagnosis of
  age and, 26
  body mass index and, 26
 glucose control in, cardiovascular events and, 13
 hepatitis C virus and, 29
 insulin therapy in, 229
 lipoprotein patterns in, 175-176
 morbid events in, 18
 pathogenesis of
  β-cell dysfunction in, 30
  insulin resistance in, 29-30
  vasodilation in, 48, *50*
 prevention of
  diet in, 210-211, 212t, 213
  exercise in, 213-216, 215t-216t
  lifestyle and drugs in, 208, 210
 prognosis in, 251, 256
 progression to in hypertension, ACE inhibitors and, 48-49, *50-51*
 undiagnosed, 27-28
  complications and, 25
  criteria for diabetic testing in, 27t
Diabetes Prevention Program (DPP), 210
Diabetic retinopathy. See *Retinopathy*.
Diagnostic criteria for diabetes, 27-28, 28t
Dialysis, ACE inhibitors and, 102t
Diastolic relaxation, cardiac RAAS expression and, 75
Diet. See also *Weight loss*.
 ADA recommendations on, 193, 213
 AHA recommendations on, 193
 alcohol in, 143, 143t, 212t, 249, 252t
 calcium in, 143t
 caloric intake in, to maintain or lose weight, 146, 148t
 carbohydrates in, 146, 211, 212t, 213
 cholesterol in, 178t, 212t, 252t
 for diabetic hypertensives, 146-147
 fads in, 211, 213
 fat in, 146-147, 178t, 210, 212t, 252t
 fiber in, 210, 212t

Diet *(continued)*
  for lipid disorders in diabetes, 178t
  potassium in, 143t
  protein in, 146, 212t, 213
  salt in, 143, 143t, 147, 149, 149t, 212t, 252t
    foods to avoid, 149t
    recommendations for, 149, 177, 178t
  sweeteners in, 212t
  vegetarian, 143t
  vitamins and minerals in, 212t, 230
  for weight loss, 146, 148t, 211, 213
Dietary Approaches to Stop Hypertension (DASH) eating plan, 145t, 150
DIGAMI trial, 245
Dihydropyridine calcium antagonists, 107. See also specific drugs.
Diltiazem, 86t, 111
Diovan. See *Valsartan.*
Diovan HCT (valsartan/hydrochlorothiazide), 169t
Dippers, 53, *54.* See also *Nondippers.*
Dipstick test, 36t, 67, 70t
Diupres (reserpine/chlorthalidone), 170t
Diuretics. See also specific drugs.
  ACE inhibitors with, 152, 166, 168t
  adverse effects of, 159t
  ARBs with, 168t-169t
  β-blockers with, 169t
    ACE inhibitors vs, 101-102, 109t, 109-110, *114,* 115t
    effectiveness of, 88, 98-99, *114,* 132t, *140,* 163, 166, 169t
  dosage of, 159t
  effectiveness of, 88, 89-99, *114,* 132t, *140,* 159t, 163, 166, 169t
  glucose metabolism and, 78, 80t-81t
  new-onset diabetes and, 78, 100
  safety of, 15, 98-100
  studies of, 158
DPP, 210
Dyazide (triamterene/hydrochlorothiazide), 170t
Dyslipidemia. See also *Lipoprotein(s).*
  atherosclerosis and, 56, 176-177
  as cardiovascular risk factor, 25, 39
  diabetes and, 55-56, 61
  in hypertension, 47t, 47-48
  stroke and, 244
  treatment of
    in diabetes, 177-178, 178t
    drugs in, 180-181, 182t, 185, *185,* 187, *188-189,* 191-192, *192,* 195t, 196
    guidelines for, 195t
    nutrition in, 195t, 212t
    order of priorities in, 197t
    physical activity in, 192
    weight loss in, 192-193, 197t

Early Treatment Diabetic Retinopathy Study (ETDRS), 204
Effect of an Angiotensin-converting Enzyme Inhibitor on Diabetic Nephropathy trial, 101, 103t
Elderly patients. See also *Systolic Hypertension in the Elderly Program (SHEP).*
  cognition and prognosis in, on SCOPE, 83t, 87t
  diuretics and glucose metabolism in, in EWPHE, 80t
  exercise in, 214-215
Enalapril (Vasotec). See also *Appropriate Blood Pressure Control in Diabetes (ABCD) trial; Fosinopril vs Amlodipine Cardiovascular Event Trial (FACET).*
  action mechanisms of, 154t
  adverse reactions to, 154t
  candesartan with, 155

Enalapril *(continued)*
  cardiovascular events and, 105t, 132t-133t
  for diabetic hypertensive patients, calcium channel blockers vs, 104-106, 105t
  dosage of, 116t, 154t
  felodipine with (Lexxel), 169t
  nitrendipine vs, 132t-133t
Enalapril/hydrochlorothiazide (Vaseretic), *140-141,* 168t
Endometrial cancer risk, 237
Endothelial cell matrix, production of, 58
Endothelial dysfunction
  adhesion of monocytes, platelets, and neutrophils in, 57-58
  atherogenesis from, 57-58
  cardiovascular disease and, 57
  causes of, 57
  hyperglycemia and, 57
  microalbuminuria and, 62, 62t
  nitric oxide and, 56, 79
  proteinuria as marker for, 62-63
  RAAS blockade and, 104
Endothelin dysfunction
  ACE inhibitors and, 79
  diabetic hypertension and, 55
Enduron (methyclothiazide), 159t
Epidemiology of diabetes, United Kingdom prospective study of, *23*
Eprosartan (Teveten), 157t
Eprosartan/hydrochlorothiazide (Teveten HCT), 168t
Estrogen
  cardioprotection from, 38
  diabetes and, 38
  replacement of, 38, 237, 255t
  study of, 237
ETDRS, 204
Ethnicity. See *Race/ethnicity;* specific ethnic group.
EURODIAB Controlled Trial of Lisinopril in Insulin-dependent Diabetes Mellitus (EUCLID), 65
European Working Party on High Blood Pressure in the Elderly (EWPHE), diuretics and glucose metabolism on, 80t
EXCEL study, 200t
Exercise
  abdominal obesity and, after menopause, 46
  aerobic, 213
  in dyslipidemia treatment, 192
  in elderly people, 214-215
  flexibility stretching in, 214-215
  guidelines for, 216t
  hypoglycemia and, 215
  precautions in diabetics, 214, 215t
  recommendations for, 145t, 254t
  in retinopathy, 214, 215t
  timing of, 216
Exercise stress test, 214
Extracellular matrix, in proteinuria and atherosclerosis, 64
Eye disease, hypertension and, 14
Ezetimibe (Zetia), 182t
Ezetimibe/simvastatin (Vytorin), 184t

FACET. See *Fosinopril vs Amlodipine Cardiovascular Event Trial.*
Family history
  of cardiovascular disease, 39, 171
  of diabetes, diabetes testing in, 27t
  of hypertension with metabolic abnormalities, 47
  of insulin resistance and microalbuminuria, 65
Fasting lipid profile, 176

Fasting plasma glucose, 172
  definition of, 27, 28t
  elevated on prior testing, 27t
Fat intake, 178t, 210, 212t, 252t
Fatty acids, free
  in insulin resistance, 45, 78, 213
  vasodilation impairment and, 46
Felodipine, 119, 133t
Felodipine/enalapril (Lexxel), 169t
Fenofibrate (Tricor)
  added to statin, 180, 192, 197t
  coronary lesion progression and, 191
  dosage and availability of, 182t, 191
  effects on lipids, 191, *192*
    in diabetes, 179
  indications for, 196, 197t
  myositis from, 197t
  studies of, 179, 191, *192*, 198t
Fiber intake, 210, 212t
Fibrates. See also specific drugs.
  dosage and availability of, 182t
  in dyslipidemia treatment, 197t
  glycemic control and, 194
  HDL level and, 194
  with HMG-CoA reductase inhibitors, 253t
  studies of, 196
Fibrinogen concentration, 58, 58t
  abdominal obesity and, 26t
  ACE inhibitors and, 79
  in hypertension, 47
Fibrinolysis, 39
Fibrosis, cardiac RAAS expression and, 75
Fish oil
  dietary, 143t
  dosage of, 183t
Flexibility stretching, 214-215
Fluid retention, 55
Fluvastatin (Lescol, Lescol XL)
  action mechanisms of, 180
  dosage and availability of, 183t
  effects on lipids, 199t
Foam cell accumulation, 64
Foot of diabetic
  proper care of, 218
  symptoms of problems in, 219t
Fosinopril (Monopril)
  action mechanisms of, 154t
  adverse reactions to, 154t
  amlodipine with, *167*
  cardiovascular events and, 106t, 132t, *167*
  dosage of, 154t
Fosinopril/hydrochlorothiazide (Monopril HCT), 168t
Fosinopril vs Amlodipine Cardiovascular Event Trial (FACET), 104-106, 106t
  ACE inhibitors in, 152, 166-167, *167*
  calcium channel blockers and, 106, 167, *167*
  design of, 85
  overall results of, 85, 132t, 167, 171
  RAAS inhibitors on, 152
4S. See *Scandinavian Simvastatin Survival Study.*
Framingham Study, 38, 245
Furosemide, 107

Gemfibrozil (Lopid)
  in diabetic dyslipidemia, 179
  dosage and availability of, 182t
  effects on lipids, 198t
  in Helsinki Heart Study, 196, 198t
  myositis from, 197t
  statins with, 181
  studies of, 198t
  for triglyceride lowering, 180, 197t
  in VA-HIT, 181, 198t
GEMINI
  design of, 160-161
  outcome of, 162t, 163
Gender. See also *Men; Menopause; Women.*
  diabetes prevalence and, 19, 22
Genetic markers of type 1 diabetes, 21
Genetics
  in diabetes, 21, 24, 27t
  in hypertension, 60
    with metabolic abnormalities, 47-48
  in insulin resistance and microalbuminuria, 65
Glinides, 223t. See also specific drugs.
Glipizide (Glucotrol)
  action mechanism of, 220
  dosage of, 222t
  renal function and, 220-221
  weight gain and, 220
Glipizide/metformin (Metaglip), 224t
Glomerular damage, diabetic, mechanisms of, 60-61
Glucophage. See *Metformin.*
Glucose control. See *Glycemic control.*
Glucose level in plasma. See *Plasma glucose.*
Glucose load, plasma glucose after, 27, 28t
Glucose metabolism
  diuretics and, 78, 80t-81t
  measurement with insulin clamp technique, 65
Glucose tolerance, impaired, in metabolic syndrome, 40t. See also *Insulin resistance.*
  hypertension and, 46
  pathophysiology of, 23-24
  on prior testing, 27t
  progression to diabetes, 24
Glucose tolerance test, oral, 28t
Glucotrol. See *Glipizide.*
Glucovance (glyburide/metformin), 224t
Glyburide (DiaBeta, Glynase PresTab, Micronase), 222t, 231
Glyburide/metformin (Glucovance), 224t
Glycation, physiology of, 208
Glycemic control
  cardiovascular events and, marginal success of, 13
  creatinine clearance and, 68
  hypertension importance over, 120-121
  microvascular complications and, 13-14
  steps in, 253t
  weight gain and, 14
Glycemic Effects in Diabetes Mellitus: Carvedilol-Metoprolol Comparison in Hypertensives (GEMINI)
  design of, 160-161, 162t, 163
  outcome of, 162t
Glycemic goals, in diabetes, 209t
Glycooxidation, cell death and, 58
Glycosylated hemoglobin. See *Hemoglobin A_{IC}.*
Glynase PresTab (glyburide), 222t, 231

Glyset (miglitol)
  action mechanism of, 229
  dosage of, 223t-224t
  side effects of, 229
GPIIb/IIA receptor antagonists, 205

Hands, cold/numb, 98, 99t
HAPPHY, on diuretics and glucose metabolism, 80t
HDFP. See *Hypertension Detection Follow-up Program.*
Health care resources, diabetic complications and, 20, 207
Heart, RAAS and, 57, 75
Heart and Estrogen/Progestin Replacement Study (HERS), 237
Heart Attack Primary Prevention in Hypertension (HAPPHY), on diuretics and glucose metabolism, 80t
Heart failure
  chronic hyperglycemia and, 19
  congestive
    aldosterone and, 246
    ARBs and, 125
    death from, 33
    in diabetes, 245-246
    simvastatin and, *190*
  systolic blood pressure and, 16
  thiazolidinediones in, 228
  in type 2 diabetes, 18
Heart Outcomes Prevention Evaluation (HOPE)
  ACE inhibition in
    in combination therapy, 79
    in diabetic hypertensive patients, 79, 85, 131, 152
    new-onset diabetes on, 76, 82t, 152-153
  angiotensin II and insulin action on, 48
  aspirin therapy in, 204, 243
  cardiovascular and renal results of, 129, 131, 131t
  size and procedures in, 82t, 85, 129
  stroke prevention in diabetics in, 242-243
Heart Outcomes Prevention Evaluation and Microalbuminuria, Cardiovascular, and Renal Outcomes study (MICRO-HOPE), 76-77
Heart Protection Study (HPS)
  design of, 178-179, 187
  dyslipidemia on, 196, 198t, 244
  results of, 179, 187, *190*
Helsinki Heart Study, 181, 196, 198t
Hemodynamics, in hypertension, 51, 53t, *54,* 55
Hemoglobin A_{IC}, 59
  ACE inhibitors and, 77
  goals for, 209t
  metoprolol vs carvedilol effect on, 161
  microvascular complication progression and, 208
Hepatitis C virus, diabetes mellitus type 2 and, 29
HERS, 237
High-density lipoprotein (HDL) cholesterol
  abdominal obesity and, 26t
  coronary heart disease and, 235
  diabetes testing and, 27t
  in hypertension, 47, 47t
  before and after menopause, 235
  in metabolic syndrome, 40t
  microalbuminuria and, 62, 62t
  raising of
    goal in, 253t
    priorities in, 197t
  in type 2 diabetes, 175

Hispanic population
  diabetes in
    prevalence of, 20, 24-25
    testing for, 27t
  increase in, 20
HMG-CoA reductase (3-hydroxy-3-methylglutaryl coenzyme A) inhibitors, 147·
    See also specific drugs.
  action mechanisms of, 180
  ADA recommendations on, 244
  in combination therapy, 180, 197t
    myositis from, 197t
  diabetes and, on CARE study, 181, 185, 187, 196, 198t
  dosage and availability of, 182t
  effectiveness of, 177
  effects on lipids, 197t
  fenofibrate with, 197t
Home measurement, of blood pressure, 141, 173, 252t
HOPE. See *Heart Outcomes Prevention Evaluation.*
Hormone replacement therapy
  cardiovascular risk and, 237, 255t
  contraindications for, 38
  in diabetic women, 237
HOT. See *Hypertension Optimal Treatment Trial.*
HPS. See *Heart Protection Study.*
Hydralazine
  added to chlorthalidone, 92
  in combination therapy, 102
  on HDFP trial, 100
  safety in diabetics, 100
Hydrochlorothiazide (HydroDIURIL, Microzide)
  ACE inhibitors with, 111, 161
  cardiovascular events and, 114t
  in combination therapy, 168t-170t
  diltiazem with/without, captopril vs, *94,* 95t, 901
  dosage of, 116, 137t, 156, 159t
  in GEMINI study, 162t
  indications for, *140*
  in MIDAS trial, 132t
  nitrendipine with/without, 94-95, 115t
  in Syst-Eur, 133t
  in VALUE study, 156
HydroDIURIL. See *Hydrochlorothiazide.*
Hydropres (reserpine/hydrochlorothiazide), 170t
Hygroton. See *Chlorthalidone.*
Hypercoagulability. See also *Blood coagulation abnormalities.*
  cardiovascular disease and, 39
  as contraindication for hormone replacement therapy, 38
  in diabetes, 13, 59-60
  in hypertension, 47
Hyperglycemia
  and congestive heart failure in diabetes, 245
  endothelial dysfunction and, 57
  organ failure and, 19
  without clinical symptoms, 23
Hyperinsulinemia
  elevated blood pressure and, mechanics of, 51-52
  visceral obesity and, 26t
Hyperkalemia, 102t
Hyperlipidemia. See also *Dyslipidemia.*
  in diabetes, 13
  frequency of, 16
  obesity incidence in, 146
  treatment priorities in, 197t

Hypertension. See also *Blood pressure.*
  abdominal obesity and, 26t
  aspirin therapy and, 47, 120, 204, 251
  cardiovascular disease and, 39-42, *41*
  clotting disorders in, 13, 47
  control of, myths and misconceptions in, 14-15
  definition of, 14
  in diabetes, 13, 39, 48-49, *50,* 51, 53, 55, 63, 78, 88. See also specific drugs and drug types.
    age and, 47-48
    autonomic neuropathy in, 53
    drugs for
      effectiveness for stroke vs coronary heart disease, 152-153
      frequency of, 14
      initial, ADA recommendations on, 155, 194
      timing of, 150
    lifestyle modifications for, 15-16, 122, 143, 145t
    management algorithm for, *140*
    predisposition to, 49, 51
    sexual dysfunction in, 17
    silent myocardial infarctions in, 17
    stroke and, 242
  diabetes testing and, 27t
  drugs for
    combinations of, 76-77. See also specific drugs and drug types.
    in diabetes, 155, 194
  dyslipidemia and, 47, 47t
  eye disease and, 14
  family history of, 47
  genetic predisposition to, 60
  glomerular capillary, 60-61
  glucose intolerance and, 46
  hemodynamic characteristics in, 51, 53t, *54,* 55
  importance over glycemic control, 120-121
  insulin resistance in, pathogenesis of, 48-49, *50-51*
  lifestyle modifications in, 122, 143, 145t
  lipoprotein abnormalities in, 47t, 47-48
  metabolic abnormalities with, 47
  nephropathy synergy with, 60
  onset of, age at, 47-48
  and progression from impaired glucose tolerance to diabetes, 24, 49, *51*
  renal artery atherosclerosis and, 142
  renal disease and, 14, 55, 60, 75-76, 101-102, 142
  as risk factor, 25
  skeletal muscle blood flow in, 46-47
  stroke and, 33
  systolic
    diabetic complications and, 49, *53*
    in elderly. See *Systolic Hypertension in the Elderly Program (SHEP).*
    isolated, 114-117
      trials of, 132t-133t
    microalbuminuria and, 62t, 64
  vascular resistance in, 55
Hypertension Detection Follow-up Program (HDFP)
  design of and patient selection for, 92-93, 98
  diuretics and glucose metabolism on, 80t
  mortality and morbidity on, 100
  stepped-care in, 92-93, 93t
Hypertension Optimal Treatment (HOT) trial
  aspirin therapy in, 120, 204
  calcium channel blockers in, 163
  diastolic blood pressure level on, 118-119, 122
  focus of, 118

Hypertension Optimal Treatment (HOT) trial *(continued)*
  goals of, 117-118
  importance of hypertension over glycemic control in, 120-121
  procedures in, 119, *120*
  results of
    cardiovascular, 119, *121*
    in diabetic vs nondiabetic participants, 119-121, *121*
    in tight vs less tight blood pressure groups, 133t
  size of, 117, 119
Hypertension studies, diabetic patient exclusion from, 91
Hypertriglyceridemia. See also *Triglycerides*.
  causes of, 176
  glycemic control and, 175
  treatment of, 197t
Hypoglycemia, 14, 215
Hypotension, postural (orthostatic), 17, 36, 53t, 55
Hyzaar (losartan/hydrochlorothiazide), *141*, 168t

IDNT. See *Irbesartan Diabetic Nephropathy Trial*.
Indapamide (Losol), 159t
Inderal LA (propranolol LA), 164t
Inderide LA (extended release propranolol/hydrochlorothiazide), 169t
Inhibitor C-reactive protein, 26t
InnoPran LX (propranolol XL), 164t
INSIGHT, 83t, 86t
Insulin clamp technique, 65
Insulin-dependent diabetes mellitus, 21
Insulin resistance. See also *Glucose tolerance, impaired*.
  abdominal obesity and, 26t, 45
  ACE inhibitors and, 76-78, 152-153
  angiotensin II and, 48, *50,* 75
  angiotensin II receptors and, 75
  in cardiometabolic syndrome, 29, 51
  causes of, 30
  in diabetes type 2 pathogenesis, 29-30
  diuretic and β-blocker effects on, 15
  family history of, 65
  free fatty acids in, 45, 78, 213
  in hypertension, 48-49, *50-51*
  microalbuminuria and, 62t, 65
  as risk factor, 25
  in skeletal muscle, 45
Insulin Resistance Atherosclerosis Study (IRAS), 29, 176-177
Insulin secretion
  absolute deficiency of, 21
  compensatory, 48
  by β-cells, 21, 23
  sulfonylurea stimulation of, 220-221
Insulin signaling, RAAS and, 75
Insulin therapy
  indications for, *227,* 229-230
  in UKPDS, 231-232
  weight gain in, 175, 232
Intermediate-density lipoprotein (IDL), in type 2 diabetes, 175
International Nifedipine Gastrointestinal Therapeutic System Study (INSIGHT), 83t, 86t
International Verapamil SR/Trandolapril (INVEST) study, 83t, 86t
Intracellular junction weakening, 58
INVEST study, 83t, 86t
IRAS, 176-177
Irbesartan (Avapro)
  action mechanisms of, 157t
  adverse reactions to, 157t

Irbesartan (Avapro) *(continued)*
  dosage of, 125-127, *128, 141,* 157t
  microproteinuria and, 155
  renal disease and, 123, 125-127
Irbesartan Diabetic Nephropathy Trial (IDNT)
  ARB effectiveness on, 68, 104, 155, 239
  design and size of, 125
  patients reaching primary end points on, 125, *126*
  RAAS inhibitors vs calcium channel blockers on, 126-127
Irbesartan/hydrochlorothiazide (Avalide), *141,* 168t
Irbesartan Microalbuminuria Type 2 Diabetes Mellitus in Hypertension Patients (IRMA 2) trial
  ARBs on, 68, 104, 123, 155
  progression to renal disease on, 127, *128,* 239
  size and design of, 126-127
IRMA 2. See *Irbesartan Microalbuminuria Type 2 Diabetes Mellitus in Hypertension Patients trial.*
Ischemic heart disease
  microalbuminuria and, *61, 62*
  undiagnosed type 2 diabetes and, 28
Isradipine, 132t

J-curve, 121
Joint National Committees on Prevention, Evaluation, Detection, and Treatment of High Blood Pressure
  JNC 6
    on blood pressure goals, 120
    on RAAS inhibitors, 114
  JNC 7
    on ARBs as initial therapy, 155
    on blood pressure goals, 120, 142, 150
    on combination therapy in diabetic hypertensives, 145, 150, 171
    on initiating drug therapy in diabetic hypertensives, 150, 252t
    on lifestyle modifications, 143t, 145t
    on microalbuminuria and rigorous blood pressure control, 142
    on RAAS inhibitors, 114
    on risk stratification, 144t

Kidney transplantation, 102t

Lactic acidosis, 225, 228
Laser photocoagulation, for retinopathy and macular edema, 35-36, 217
Left ventricular function, ACE inhibitors and, 75
Left ventricular hypertrophy
  abdominal obesity and, 26t
  nighttime blood pressure and, 53, 55
  regression of, 127
Leg pain, 215
Lescol (fluvastatin)
  action mechanisms of, 180
  dosage and availability of, 182t
  effects on lipids, 199t
Levatol (penbutolol), 165t
Lexxel (felodipine/enalapril), 169t
LIFE. See *Losartan Intervention for Endpoint Reduction in Hypertension study.*
Life expectancy in diabetes, 18-19, *24*
Lifestyle modifications
  antihypertensive agents and, 122, 143
  in diabetic hypertensive patient, 15-16, 145t
  examples of, 143, 143t, 145t
  in type 2 diabetes prevention, 208-216

Lipid lowering drugs
  action mechanisms of, 180
  clinical trials of, 181, 185, 187, 191-192
  liver function and, 180
Lipid profile, fasting, 176
Lipid Research Clinics Follow-up Study, 235
LIPID trial
  mortality and nonfatal myocardial infarctions in, 181, 186t
  size of and patient selection for, 187
Lipitor (atorvastatin)
  clinical study of, 187
  dosage and availability of, 182t, 199t
  effects on lipids, 199t
Lipoprotein(s). See also *High-density lipoprotein cholesterol; Hyperlipidemia; Low-density lipoprotein; Very low-density lipoprotein.*
  abnormalities in. See *Dyslipidemia.*
  cardiovascular disease and, 39
  diuretic and β-blocker effects on, 15
  oxidation of, in hypertension, 47t
  patterns of, in type 2 diabetes, 175
Lipoprotein (a), 58t, 58-59
Lipoprotein lipase
  hepatic, LDL and HDL particle alteration by, 186
  in hypertension, 47t
Lisinopril (Prinivil, Zestril)
  action mechanisms of, 154t
  adverse reactions to, 154t
  clinical trials of, 77
  dosage of, *140,* 154t
  effectiveness of, 77
  indications for, *140*
Lisinopril/hydrochlorothiazide (Prinzide, Zestoretic), *140,* 168t
Lispro, 229
Liver, insulin resistance in, 29
Liver function, lipid-lowering drugs and, 180
Long-Term Intervention with Pravastatin in Ischaemic Disease (LIPID) trial
  mortality and nonfatal myocardial infarctions in, 181, 186t
  size of and patient selection for, 187
Lopid. See *Gemfibrozil.*
Lopressor. See *Metoprolol* entries.
Losartan (Cozaar). See also *Reduction of Endpoints in Noninsulin-dependent Diabetes Mellitus with an Angiotensin II Antagonist (RENAAL) trial.*
  action mechanisms of, 157t
  adverse reactions to, 157t
  dosage of, 123, *141,* 157t
  indications for, *140-141*
  microproteinuria and, 155
  renal disease and, 123-124, *124*
Losartan/hydrochlorothiazide (Hyzaar), *141,* 168t
Losartan Intervention for Endpoint Reduction in Hypertension (LIFE) study
  ARBs in diabetics vs nondiabetics on, 129
  ARBs vs ACE inhibitors on, 156
  ARBs vs other therapies on, 87t
  losartan vs atenolol on, 128-129, *130*
  new-onset diabetes on, 83t, 87t
  size of and drugs in, 83t
Losol (indapamide), 159t
Lotensin (benazepril), 154t
Lotensin HCT (benazepril/hydrochlorothiazide), 168t
Lotrel (amlodipine/benazepril), 169t
Lovastatin (Altocor, Mevacor)
  action mechanisms of, 180
  and cardiovascular disease reduction in diabetics, 187

Lovastatin (Altocor, Mevacor) *(continued)*
　dosage and availability of, 183t
　effects on lipids, 199t-200t
　niacin with (Advicor), 184t
Low-density lipoprotein (LDL)
　in hypertension, 47t, 47-48
　lowering of
　　with HMG-CoA reductase inhibitor, 172
　　priorities in, 197t
　before and after menopause, 235
　oxidation of
　　ACE inhibitors and, 79
　　in proteinuria and atherosclerosis, 64
　in type 2 diabetes, 175
Low-density lipoprotein (LDL) cholesterol, calculation of, 176

Macular edema, 35-36, 217
Mavik. See *Trandolapril*.
Maxzide (triamterene/hydrochlorothiazide), 146t
MDRD trial, 238
Medical Research Council, on diuretics and glucose metabolism, 80t
Meglitinide, 221, 223t
　dosage of, 223t
　indications for, 226
Men, microalbuminuria in, 62t
Menopause. See also *Women*.
　age-related abdominal obesity after, 46
　cardiovascular disease after, 38, 235
Mesangial proliferation, in proteinuria and atherosclerosis, 64
Mesenteric fat. See *Abdominal obesity*.
Metabolic syndrome (syndrome X)
　clinical features of, 39-40, 40t
　microalbuminuria in, 62, 62t
　RAAS inhibitors for, 79
　risk criteria in, 40t
Metaglip (glipizide/metformin), 224t
Metformin (Glucophage)
　action mechanism of, 225
　in combination therapy, 171, 221
　contraindications to, 225, *227,* 228
　diabetes development slowed by, 26, 210
　dosage of, 223t
　effectiveness of, 232
　glipizide with (Metaglip), 224t
　glyburide with (Glucovance), 224t
　half-life of, 223t
　hypoglycemia with, 232
　indications for, 171, 225, *226-227,* 228
　lactic acidosis and, 225, 228
　rosiglitazone with (Avandamet), 224t
　thiazolidinediones with, 228
　in UKPDS, 231-232
　weight gain and, 225, 232
Metformin/sulfonylurea, 171
Methyclothiazide (Enduron), 159t
Methyldopa/hydrochlorothiazide (Aldoril), 170t
Metolazone (Mykrox, Zaroxolyn), 159t
Metoprolol (Lopressor). See also *Glycemic Effects in Diabetes Mellitus: Carvedilol-Metoprolol Comparison in Hypertensives (GEMINI)*.
　action mechanisms of, 164t
　carvedilol vs, 160-151, 162t, 163
　dosage of, 160-161, 164t
　HbA_{1C} and, 161

Metoprolol/hydrochlorothiazide (Lopressor HCT), 169t
Metoprolol XR (Toprol-XL), 164t
Mevacor. See *Lovastatin.*
Micardis (telmisartan), 157t
Micardis HCT (telmisartan/hydrochlorothiazide), 169t
Micral test, 36t
MICRO-HOPE (Heart Outcomes Prevention Evaluation and Microalbuminuria, Cardiovascular, and Renal Outcomes study), 76-77, 242-243
Microalbuminuria
  abdominal obesity and, 26t
  cardiovascular risks and, 25, 62, 62t, 68, *69,* 142
  as consequence of hypertension and diabetes, 60-62
  definition of, 36t, 61
  endothelial dysfunction and, 62, 62t
  family history of, 65, 67
  hypertension and
    control of, 142
    systolic, 64-65
  insulin resistance and, 62t, 65
  ischemic heart disease risk and, *61,* 62
  nighttime blood pressure and, 53, 61, 62t
  oxidative stress and, 62, 62t
  renal disease progression and, 66-68
  treatment of, 37
Micronase (glyburide), 222t, 231
Microproteinuria, 70t
  ARBs and, 70t, 126-127
  irbesartan and, 127, *128*
Microzide. See *Hydrochlorothiazide.*
MIDAS analysis, 132t
Miglitol (Glyset)
  action mechanism of, 229
  dosage of, 223t-224t
  side effects of, 229
Mineral intake, 212t, 230
Minizide (prazosin/polythiazide), 170t
Modified Dietary Protein in Renal Disease (MDRD) trial, 238
Moduretic (amiloride/hydrochlorothiazide), 170t
Moexipril (Univasc), 154t
Moexipril/hydrochlorothiazide (Uniretic), 168t
Monocytes, adhesion to endothelium, 57-58
Monopril. See *Fosinopril* entries.
Morning urine protein, 67
Motion exercise, 213-214
MRC, on diuretics and glucose metabolism, 80t
MRFIT. See *Multiple Risk Factor Intervention Trial.*
Multiple Risk Factor Intervention Trial (MRFIT), design of, 40
  in diabetics vs nondiabetics, 40-41, *41*
  diuretics on, 80t
Muscular hypertrophy, RAAS blockade and, 104
Mykrox (metolazone), 159t
Myocardial infarction. See also *Cardiovascular disease/events.*
  death from
    in diabetes, 33, *130,* 131t
    in women, 38
  nonfatal, on CARE study, 186t
  ramipril and, 79
  risk of, in diabetic vs nondiabetic population, 34, *35*
  silent, 17, 236
  simvastatin and, *190*
Myocardial Infarction Data Acquisition System (MIDAS) analysis, 132t
Myositis, 197t

Nadolol (Corgard)
   action mechanism of, 164t
   diuretic with, *141*
   dosage of, 164t
   indications for, *141*
Nadolol/bendroflumethiazide (Corzide), *141,* 169t
Nateglinide (Starlix)
   action mechanism of, 221, 225
   dosage of, 223t
   metformin with, 225
   pharmacokinetics of, 223t, 225
National Cholesterol Education Program (NCEP) recommendations
   dietary, 177, 178t
   on lipid levels, 194, 195t, 196
National Kidney Foundation recommendations for blood pressure
   in diabetics, 120, 150
   in nondiabetics, 120
Native Americans, diabetes in
   prevalence of, 24
   testing for, 27t
NCEP recommendations
   dietary, 177, 178t
   on lipid levels, 194, 195t, 196
Nephropathy
   in diabetes, 18, 36-37, 76
      mechanisms of, 60
   hypertension synergy with, 60
Neuropathy, diabetic
   autonomic
      in hypertension, 17
      nondipping and, 53
   orthostatic hypotension as, 36
Neutrophils, adhesion to endothelium, 58
Niacin
   in diabetes, 252t
   effects on lipids, 180, 197t-198t
   side effects of, 180
Niacin/lovastatin (Advicor), 184t
Nicotinic acid (Niacor, Niaspan, Slo-Niacin)
   in diabetic dyslipidemia management, 197t-198t
   dosage of, 182t-183t
   statins with, myositis from, 197t
Nifedipine, 107
   on INSIGHT study, 83t, 86t
Nisoldipine
   cardiovascular events and, 105t, 132t
   enalapril vs, 104, 105t, 132t
Nitrendipine, 115-116, 116t, 133t. See also *Systolic Hypertension Trial in Europe (Syst-Eur) trial.*
Nitric oxide
   abnormal vascular metabolism of, 56
   endothelial dysfunction and, 56, 79
   metabolism of, cardiac RAAS expression and, 75
   platelet production of, 59t
   vasorelaxation response to, 53t
Non-insulin-dependent diabetes. See *Diabetes mellitus type 2.*
Nondippers, 53, *54*
   inaccuracy of daytime blood pressure readings in, 141
   left ventricular hypertrophy and, 53, 55
   microalbuminuria and, 53, 61, 62t
   office blood pressure measurement in, 139, 141
Norepinephrine, 55
Number necessary to treat to prevent one cardiovascular event, 181, 182t-183t

Obesity. See also *Weight gain; Weight loss.*
  abdominal
    age-related, 42, 46
    exercise and, after menopause, 46
    hypertension and, 26t
    insulin resistance and, 26t, 45
    metabolic and cardiovascular risk factors and, 25, 26t
    microalbuminuria and, 62t
  blood pressure cuff in, 139
  cardiovascular disease and, 39, 42
  in diabetes, 13, 19, 146
  diabetes testing in, 27t
  exercise and, 46
  insulin resistance in, 29
  microalbuminurea and, 62t
  prevalence of, 16, 20, *25*
    in diabetics and hyperlipidemia, 146
    and progression from impaired glucose tolerance to diabetes, 23-24, *25,* 26t
  in women, 236
Olmesartan (Benicar), 157t, 169t
Omental fat. See *Abdominal obesity.*
Oral glucose tolerance test, 28t
Organ failure, chronic hyperglycemia and, 19
Orinase (tolbutamide)
  action mechanism of, 220
  dosage of, 222t
Orthostatic hypotension, 17, 36, 53t, 55
Oslo study, diuretics and glucose metabolism on, 80t
Oxidation, of lipoproteins, in hypertension, 47t
Oxidative stress
  microalbuminuria and, 62, 62t
  vascular
    cardiovascular disease and, 39
    nitric oxide metabolism and, 56
Oxygen free radicals
  excess generation of, 57
  microalbuminuria and, 62, 62t

Pain, resting, in feet, 219t
Pancreas, worn out, 48
Pathophysiology of diabetes
  type 1, 20-21
  type 2, 21, 23
Penbutolol (Levatol), 165t
PEPI, 237
Perindopril (Aceon), 154t
Peripheral antiadrenergic agents, hyperglycemia risk with, *161*
Peripheral vascular disease
  amputation in, 218
  in diabetes, death from, 33
  prevention of, 218, 219t
  undiagnosed type 2 diabetes and, 28
Peripheral vascular resistance, in hypertensive diabetics, 53t
D-Phenylalanine derivative, 223t
Photocoagulation with laser, for retinopathy and macular edema, 35-36, 217
Physical inactivity. See *Exercise; Sedentary lifestyle.*
Pindolol, 165t
Pioglitazone (Actos)
  action mechanisms of, 228
  contraindications for, 228
  dosage of, 223t
  insulin with, weight gain and, 230

Plasma glucose
  bedtime, goals for, 209t
  casual, definition of, 27, 28t
  fasting, 172
    definition of, 27, 28t
    elevated on prior testing, 27t
  after glucose load, 27
  postprandial, 27, 210
  preprandial, goals for, 209t
Plasma volume, in hypertensive diabetics, 53t
Plasminogen activator, 26t
Plasminogen activator inhibitor-1, 58t, 61
Platelet, nitric oxide production by, 59t
Platelet aggregation/adhesion
  cardiovascular disease and, 39
  in diabetes and hypertension, 59t, 59-60
  drugs for, 203-205
  endothelial, 57-58
Plavix (clopidogrel), 205
Postmenopausal Estrogen/Progestin Intervention (PEPI), 237
Postprandial plasma glucose, 27, 210
Postural hypotension, 17, 36, 53t, 55
Posture, in blood pressure measurement, 142
Potassium channel, cardiac RAAS expression and, 75
Potassium intake, 143t
Prandin. See *Repaglinide*.
Pravastatin (Pravachol)
  in cardiovascular protection, 181, 185, 187, *188-189*
  in CARE trial, 181, 185, 187
  in diabetics vs nondiabetics, 181, *188-189*
  dosage and availability of, 183t
  effects on lipids, 198t-200t
  indications for, 180
  in LIPID trial, 181, 186t
Prazosin, 107
Prazosin/polythiazide (Minizide), 170t
Precose. See *Acarbose*.
Pregnancy
  diabetic retinopathy in, 34-35
  pharmacological therapy in, *226-227*
Preprandial glucose, diabetic goals for, 209t
Prevalence of diabetes
  aging and, 20, *21*
  in America, 19
  global estimates and projections of, 19, *20*
  obesity and, 20
  race and, 19
Prevalite (cholestyramine), 182t
Prinivil. See *Lisinopril*.
Prinzide (lisinopril/hydrochlorothiazide), 168t
Progestin, 237
Propranolol (extended release)/hydrochlorothiazide (Inderide LA), 169t
Propranolol LA (Inderal LA), 164t
Propranolol XL (InnoPran XL), 164t
Prostanoids, platelet generation of, 59t
Protein C, 58t, 59
Protein intake, 212t
Protein S, 58t, 59
Proteinuria. See also *Microproteinuria*.
  albumin content in, 60
  atherosclerosis and, 64-65
  as marker for endothelial dysfunction and atherosclerosis, 62-63
  reduction of, 67

Proteinuria *(continued)*
  in renal function prognosis, 102
  systolic blood pressure and, 16
Pulse pressure, vascular rigidity and, 122

QT rate, in diabetes, 246-247
Questran/Questran Light (cholestyramine), 182t
Quinapril (Accupril), *140,* 154t

Race/ethnicity
  diabetes in
    prevalence of, 19-20, *22,* 24-25, 27t
    testing for, 27t
  kidney disease and, 238
Ramipril (Altace)
  action mechanisms of, 154t
  adverse reactions to, 154t
  cardiovascular events and, 76, 79, 129, 131t
  in diabetes, 77
  dosage of, *140,* 154t
  effectiveness of, 77
  HbA_{1C} and, 77
  in HOPE study, 129
  indications for, *140*
  renal effects of, 131
Randomized Evaluation of Strategies for Left Ventricular Dysfunction (RESOLV), 155
Reduction of Endpoints in Noninsulin-dependent Diabetes Mellitus with an Angiotensin II Antagonist, Losartan (RENAAL) trial
  ARBs and renal disease progression on, 68, 155, 239
  design and size of, 123-125
  diabetic nephropathy and, 104, 123, *124*
Referred care antihypertensive regimen, in HDFP, 92-93, 93t
REGRESS, 200t
Relaxation techniques, 143t
RENAAL. See *Reduction of Endpoints in Noninsulin-dependent Diabetes Mellitus with an Angiotensin II Antagonist, Losartan trial.*
Renal artery atherosclerosis, 142
Renal disease
  ACE inhibitors and, 75-76, 101-102, 102t, 104, 131, 131t, 238-239
  amlodipine and, *124, 126,* 1125
  ARBs and, 104, 123-127, *124,* 239
  chronic hyperglycemia and, 19
  death from, 14, 38
  in diabetes, 18, 36-37, 76
  hypertension and, 14, 55, 60, 75-76, 101-102, 142
  prognosis of, proteinuria in, 102
  progression of, microalbuminuria and, 66-68
  undiagnosed type 2 diabetes and, 28-29
Renin-angiotensin-aldosterone system (RAAS)
  ACE inhibitors and, 73, 88-89
  blockade of, vascular/endothelial/muscular effects of, 104
  in cardiovascular disease, 57, 75
  functions of, 73
  hypertensive action of, 73
  inhibitors of
    calcium channel blockers vs, 152
    in combination therapy for nephropathy, 102
    new-onset diabetes and, 52
  insulin signaling and, 75
  microalbuminuria progression and, 68

Repaglinide (Prandin)
  action mechanism of, 221
  contraindications for, 221
  dosage of, 223t
  indications for, *227*
  renal function and, 221
Reserpine
  chlorthalidone with, 92, 133t, 170t
  safety of, 100
Reserpine/thiazide (Hydropres), 170t
Resistance training, precautions in, 214t
RESOLV, 155
Resting pain, 209t
Retinopathy
  blindness and, 28, 34, 217
  early manifestations of, 34
  exercise in, 214, 215t
  management of, 217
  in pregnancy, 34-35
  systolic blood pressure and, 16
  treatment of, 35-36
  in type 2 diabetes, 18
  on UKPDS, 88
Revascularization, peripheral, 218
Reye's syndrome, 204
Rosiglitazone (Avandia)
  action mechanisms of, 228
  contraindications to, 228
  dosage of, 223t
  half-life of, 223t
  weight gain and, 228
Rosiglitazone/metformin (Avandamet), 224t
Rosuvastatin (Crestor)
  in diabetics, 180
  dosage of, 183t, 199t
  effect on lipid types, 199t

Salt intake, 143, 143t, 147, 149, 149t, 212t, 252t
  foods to avoid, 149t
  recommendations for, 149, 177, 178t
Salt retention
  in diabetic nephropathy, 55
  microalbuminuria and, 62t
Salt sensitivity, in diabetics, 147
Scandinavian Simvastatin Survival Study (4S)
  coronary heart disease incidence on, 181, *185,* 196
  design of, 185
  dyslipidemia on, 198t, 244
  preventive statins on, 235
SCOPE, 83t, 87t
Sectral (acebutolol), 165t
Sedentary lifestyle
  cardiovascular disease and, 39
  diabetes prevalence and, 19, 24
Seventh Joint National Committee on Prevention, Evaluation, Detection, and Treatment of High Blood Pressure. See *Joint National Committees on Prevention, Evaluation, Detection, and Treatment of High Blood Pressure, JNC 7.*
Sexual dysfunction
  antihypertensives and, in diabetics vs nondiabetics, 98, 99t
  in hypertensive diabetic, 17
SHEP. See *Systolic Hypertension in the Elderly Program.*

Simvastatin (Zocor). See also *Scandinavian Simvastatin Survival Study (4S)*.
  in coronary protection, 179, 185, *185, 190*
  dosage and availability of, 179, 183t, 187
  effects on lipids, 180, 198t-200t
  ezetimibe with (Vytorin), 184t
  in HPS, 179, 187, *190*
Sixth Joint National Committee on Prevention, Evaluation, Detection, and Treatment of High Blood Pressure. See *Joint National Committees on Prevention, Evaluation, Detection, and Treatment of High Blood Pressure, JNC 6.*
Skeletal muscle
  age-related loss of, 42
  blood flow in, in hypertension, 46-47
  insulin resistance in, 45
  nutrient delivery to, ACE inhibitors and, 49
Skin, in diabetic foot problems, 219t
Slo-Niacin, 183t
Smoking, 13, 39
  cessation of, 143t, 254t
  diabetes synergism with, in diabetes-related death, 42
  on MRFIT, 40-41
  oxygen free radical generation and, 57
  peripheral vascular disease and, 218
  renal artery atherosclerosis and, 142
Smooth muscle hypertrophy, RAAS blockade and, 104
Sodium pump, cardiac RAAS expression and, 75
Spironolactone/hydrochlorothiazide (Aldactazide), 170t
Starlix (nateglinide)
  action mechanisms of, 221, 225
  dosage of, 223t
  metformin with, 225
  pharmacokinetics of, 223t, 225
Statins. See *HMG-CoA reductase inhibitors.*
Stepped-care antihypertensive regimen, 92-93, 93t
Steroids, and progression from impaired glucose tolerance to diabetes, 24
STOP-2, 83t, 86t, 87, 158
Stress test, exercise, 214
Stroke. See also *Cerebrovascular disease.*
  abdominal obesity and, 26t
  death from, 241
    in women, 33, 37-38, *130*, 236
  in diabetes
    incidence of, 241-242
    losartan vs atenolol and, *130*
    prevention of, 242-243
  dyslipidemia and, 244
  hypertension and, 33
  pharmacologic prevention of, 151
  systolic blood pressure and, 16
  in type 2 diabetes, 18
    undiagnosed, 28
  on UKPDS, 144, 242
Study on Cognition and Prognosis in the Elderly (SCOPE), 83t, 87t
Sudden cardiac death, in diabetes, 246-247
Sulfonylureas. See also specific drugs.
  action mechanisms of, 220, 222t
  biguanide with, 224t
  dosage of, 222t
  indications for, *226-227*
  metformin with, 171
  in UKPDS, 231-232
  weight gain and hypoglycemia with, 232
Swedish Trial in Older Patients with Hypertension-2 (STOP-2), 83, 87, 158

Sweeteners, 212t
Symptoms of diabetes, 21
Syndrome X (metabolic syndrome)
  clinical features of, 39-40, 40t
  microalbuminuria in, 62, 62t
  RAAS inhibitors for, 79
  risk criteria in, 40t
Systolic Hypertension in the Elderly Program (SHEP)
  adverse effects in, 98, 99t
  combination therapy in, 100, 116
  diabetes and cardiovascular event rates in, 94-95, 96t, *97*, 158
  in diabetics and nondiabetics, 95
  diastolic blood pressure in, 98, 118, 122
  diuretics and glucose metabolism on, 80t
  diuretics in, 80t, 94, 100, 116, 133t
  number of risk factors and therapeutic results in, 117
  overall results of, 133t, 158
  size of and patient selection in, 94, 98, 133t
  stroke prevention in, 242
Systolic Hypertension Trial in Europe (Syst-Eur)
  aggressive treatment in, 121
  calcium channel blockers in, 163
  cardiovascular event results of, 133t
  endpoints of, 132t
  multifaceted approach in, 121
  purpose of, 114-115
  size and procedures in, 115-117, 132t
  stroke prevention in diabetics in, 242

Tarka (trandolapril/extended release verapamil), 169t
Telmisartan (Micardis), 169t
Telmisartan/hydrochlorothiazide (Micardis HCT), 169t
Tenoretic (atenolol/chlorthalidone), 169t
Tenormin. See *Atenolol*.
Teveten (eprosartan), 157t
Teveten HCT (eprosartan/hydrochlorothiazide), 168t
Thalitone. See *Chlorthalidone*.
Thiazide diuretics
  dosage, adverse effects, and effectiveness of, 159t
  hyperglycemia risk with, *161*
  safety in diabetics, 100, 156, 158
Thiazolidinediones. See also specific drugs.
  action mechanism of, 228
  biguanide with, 224t
  contraindications to, 228
  diabetes development and, 26
  dosage of, 223t
  half-life of, 223t
  indications for, 220, *226-227*
  insulin with, 228
  side effects of, 228, 230
  vascular effects of, 232
Thrombin-antithrombin complexes, 58t
Thrombus formation, in hyperglycemia, 58
Ticlopidine (Ticlid), 205
Timolide (timolol/hydrochlorothiazide), 169t
Timolol (Blocadren), 164t
Timolol/hydrochlorothiazide (Timolide), 169t
Tolazamide (Tolinase)
  action mechanism of, 220
  dosage of, 222t

Tolbutamide (Orinase)
    action mechanism of, 220
    dosage of, 222t
TOMHS, 81t
Toprol-XL (metoprolol), 164t
Trandolapril (Mavik)
    action mechanism of, 154t
    adverse effects of, 154t
    dosage of, 154t
    in INVEST study, 83t-84t, 86t
Trandolapril/verapamil extended release (Tarka), 169t
Treatment of Mild Hypertension Study (TOMHS), 81t
Triamterene/hydrochlorothiazide (Dyazide, Maxzide), 170t
Tricor. See *Fenofibrate*.
Triglycerides. See also *Hypertriglyceridemia*.
    abdominal obesity and, 26t
    atherogenesis and, 56
    diabetes testing and, 27t
    goal levels of, 251, 253t
    in hypertension, 47t
    before and after menopause, 235
    in metabolic syndrome, 40t
    metabolism of, 445
    microalbuminuria and, 62t
    in type 2 diabetes, 175

UKPDS. See *United Kingdom Prospective Diabetes Study*.
Undiagnosed diabetes, 27-28
    criteria for diabetic testing in, 27t
Uniretic (moexipril/hydrochlorothiazide), 168t
United Kingdom Prospective Diabetes Study (UKPDS)
    ACE inhibitors and cardiac mortality on, 88
    atrial fibrillation in diabetes in, 243
    β-blockers in
        ACE inhibitor results vs, 85, 88, 109t, 109-110, 114
        diuretics with, 76, 158
        effectiveness of, 158, 160
        RAAS and, 88
        safety of, 110
    blood pressure control and diabetes in, *110*
    blood pressure goals in, in diabetics vs nondiabetics, 119-120
    combinations of agents in, 166
    diuretics in, 76, 158
    glycemic control and vascular events in, 231
    goals of, 107
    HbA_{1C} and complications on, 208
    hypertension importance vs glycemic control in, 121
    insulin vs sulfonylureas in, 231
    metformin in, in overweight patients, 232
    number of risk factors and therapeutic results in, 117
    overall results of, 231-232
    reduced β-cell function in, 30
    retinopathy in, 88
    size and procedures in, 107, *108,* 133t
    stroke risk in, 144, 233, 242
    sulfonylureas and insulin in, 221, 232
    three facets of, 107
    tight vs less tight blood pressure control in, 108, *108, 112-113,* 133t-134t, 231
    weight gain in, 232
Univasc (moexipril), 154t

VA-HIT. See *Veterans Affairs High-Density Lipoprotein Cholesterol Intervention Trial*.

Valsalvalike maneuvers, 215t
Valsartan (Diovan). See also *Valsartan Antihypertension Long-Term Use Evaluation (VALUE)*.
  action mechanisms of, 157t
  adverse reactions to, 157t
  amlodipine vs, 105
  dosage of, 156, 157t
  proteinuria and, 155
Valsartan Antihypertensive Long-term Use Evaluation (VALUE)
  amlodipine success on, 105
  diabetic nephropathy and congestive heart failure in, 166
  drugs used in, 83t, 87t, 105, 151, 156, 166
  goals of, 156
  insulin action and angiotensin II in, 48
  new-onset diabetes in, 151, 156
  results of, 156
  size and duration of, 83t, 87t
Valsartan/hydrochlorothiazide (Diovan HCT), 169t
VALUE. See *Valsartan Antihypertensive Long-term Use Evaluation*.
Vascular compliance, cardiovascular disease and, 39
Vascular disease. See also *Cerebrovascular disease; Peripheral vascular disease; Stroke*.
  nitric oxide metabolism and, 57
Vascular oxidative stress, cardiovascular disease and, 39
Vascular resistance, in hypertension, 55
Vascular rigidity, pulse pressure and, 122
Vaseretic (enalapril/hydrochlorothiazide), *140*, 168t
Vasoconstriction, in hypertensive diabetics, 53t
Vasodilation, free fatty acids and, 46
Vasodilators
  added to chlorthalidone, 92
  hyperglycemia risk with, *161*
  insulin resistance and, 48, 50
Vasorelaxation, in response to nitric oxide, 53t
Vasotec. See *Enalapril*.
Vegetarian diet, 143t
Ventricular arrhythmia, in diabetes, 246
Ventricular hypertrophy. See *Left ventricular hypertrophy*.
Very low-density lipoprotein (VLDL)
  in hypertension, 47, 47t
  hypertriglyceridemia and, 176
  metabolism of, in skeletal muscle, 45
  in type 2 diabetes, 175
Veterans Administration single-drug therapy for hypertension in men, 81t
Veterans Affairs High-Density Lipoprotein Cholesterol Intervention Trial (VA-HIT)
  fibrates in, 196
  gemfibrozil in, 181, 198t
  nonfatal myocardial infarctions and cardiovascular death in, 186t
Visceral fat. See *Abdominal obesity*.
Vitamin intake, 212t
Vytorin (ezetimibe/simvastatin), 184t

Walking, 214, 215t
Warfarin therapy, in diabetic stroke prevention, 243-244
Weight
  ideal, 171, 254t
    calculation of, 147t
  normal, hypertension in, 46
Weight gain
  glycemic control and, 14
  in insulin therapy, 175, 232
  metformin and, 225, 232

Weight lifting, 215t
Weight loss
  benefits of, 211
  calculating calories for, 146, 148t
  diets in, 211, 213
  exercise in, 213-214
  in hyperlipidemia, 192-193, 197t
  indications for, 143t, 145t, 145-146
  pharmacological therapy in, *226*, 253t
  rate of, 211
WelChol, 182t
Women
  age-related abdominal obesity in, 46
  aspirin therapy in, 236-237, 247
  cardiovascular disease in, 37-39
    death from, 235-236
  hormone replacement therapy in, diabetes and, 237
  obesity in, 236
  stroke in, 37-38, *130*, 236
WOSCOPS, 200t

Zaroxolyn (metolazone), 159t
Zebeta (bisoprolol)
  action mechanism of, 164t
  diuretic with, *141*
  dosage of, 164t
Zestoretic (lisinopril/hydrochlorothiazide), *140*, 168t
Zestril. See *Lisinopril*.
Zetia (ezetimibe), 182t
Ziac (bisoprolol/hydrochlorothiazide), *141*, 169t
Zocor. See *Simvastatin*.